SEPARATING TOGETHER

SEPARATING TOGETHER
How Divorce Transforms Families

ABIGAIL J. STEWART
ANNE P. COPELAND
NIA LANE CHESTER
JANET E. MALLEY
NICOLE B. BARENBAUM

THE GUILFORD PRESS
New York   London

© 1997 The Guilford Press
A Division of Guilford Publications, Inc.
72 Spring Street, New York, NY 10012

Printed in the United States of America

This book is printed on acid-free paper.

Last digit is print number: 9   8   7   6   5   4   3   2

Library of Congress Cataloging-in-Publication Data

Separating together: how divorce transforms families / Abigail J.
Stewart . . . [et al.].
    p.   cm.
Includes bibliographical references and index.
ISBN 1-57230-235-6
    1. Divorce—United States—Psychological aspects.   2. Family—
United States—Psychological aspects.   3. Divorced parents—United
States.   4. Children of divorced parents—United States.   5. Broken
homes—United States.   I. Stewart, Abigail J.
HQ834.S46   1997
306.89—dc21   97-8707
                                                                            CIP

Preface

This book is a thoroughly collaborative project. From the research project we conducted together at Boston University to the actual book writing, our goal has been a collaboration in which several voices could be distinguished, but would blend together harmoniously. In the process of writing we planned the overall structure together, shared chapters with each other, and made suggestions to each other for revisions. We periodically met as a group to redefine our collective vision. In the end, every chapter is a product of all of our work. We have, however, indicated for each chapter who drafted the chapter initially and took responsibility for subsequent revisions. We found throughout this process that our differences were always helpful to each other; we hope they make the book richer, if more complex.

Perhaps because it has been such a deeply collaborative project, the road to publication has been long. We've lived through many family—and work—transformations ourselves. Our own families have been changed by marriages, divorces, births, adoptions, and illnesses. During this period, we've had many moves among us, as well as graduations, awards of tenure, promotions, and job changes. The change that most affected this book, though, was our loss of Joseph M. Healy, Jr., as a collaborator. He was at the heart of the Family Changes Project. When his career change made it necessary for him to stop working with us on the manuscript, we celebrated his personal growth and new work satisfactions, but we have missed him. His work on the project contributed to every page of the book.

We are pleased to thank here the institutions, funding sources, and individuals who made our work on this project possible. Boston University, the Murray Research Center at Radcliffe College, and the University of Michigan all provided critical space and computer resources at various stages of the project. Several grants from the Spencer Foundation, the National Institute of

Mental Health (RO1-MH38801, RO3-MH393302, and RO3-MH38026) and the Boston University Graduate School provided financial support for the data collection. Drs. Frances Grossman and Leslie Brody provided clinical advice to the research group; Professor Michael Wheeler provided us with legal advice. Various kinds of assistance over the years were provided by Krisanne Bursik, Deborah Cohen, Elizabeth Cole, Alisa Dennis, Julie Eisenstein, Ruth Faas, Molly Fleming, Carol Franz, Susan Frazier Kouassi, Amy Harrison, Nancy Jarnis, Ann Jirkovsky, Marcia Johnston, Anne-Marie Jolly, Beth Morrow, Deborah Nelson, Carmen Peralta, Ellen Milenko Reiner, Susan Ruch, Jone Sloman, Althea Smith, Timothy Stewart-Winter, Joan Test, Elizabeth Vandewater, Patricia Waters, David G. Winter, and Nicholas J. G. Winter. Finally, many individuals provided us with editorial advice, feedback, and support. These included several people who reviewed the entire manuscript: Faye Crosby, Carol Franz, Paul Wink, David Winter, and our editor at The Guilford Press, Kitty Moore.

Most of all, we are grateful to the families who offered so much of themselves during a difficult time in their lives.

Contents

PART FOUR
PARENTAL DIVORCE AS A
FAMILY TRANSFORMATION

SEPARATING TOGETHER

PART ONE

THE PSYCHOLOGICAL EXPERIENCE OF PARENTAL DIVORCE

In this first section of the book, we examine the psychological experience of divorce. We begin by examining popular images of divorce, and compare them with the experience of three families from our study. We show that these popular images—including those psychologists share—need to be changed to incorporate the potential for personal growth, a focus on the family as a whole, and recognition of the way that gender roles change in the course of divorce.

In the second chapter, we explain how a study's design limits the questions it can answer. We describe our study's design and stress that it is focused on how different individuals and families respond to parental separation and divorce.

In the third chapter, we describe what the adult family members told us about their experience of divorce. We try to capture the texture of their experience, and we emphasize that, for parents, the separation simultaneously marks the end of a struggle to stay married and the beginning of a new family life. In the early period after the separation, parents mostly focused on handling the concrete, everyday demands of their new household, including (especially) their children. A year later they were more focused on their own personal needs and their relationships with friends and relatives.

In the fourth chapter we describe the children's experience. Again, we try to capture its texture, and show that, for them, the parental separation is mostly unexpected and unwanted, so in the early period they are simply absorbing this painful surprise. Later on the children not only report acceptance of the new family structure, and some benefits as well as losses, but are impressively aware of the differences between their own experience and that of their parents.

In comparing parents' and children's experience we found it useful to draw on a framework for understanding adaptation to life changes in general. According to this view, changes stimulate psychological reorientation and a sequence of stances toward the environment. In the beginning individuals are confused but receptive, and are searching for ways to get their needs met. Later they focus on establishing their own competence and taking initiative. We note that the physical separation initiates this reorientation for the children, but that the process starts much earlier for parents. As a result, parents and children are in very different psychological states at this point in the process of family transformations.

Taken together, these four chapters outline our perspective on parental separation and divorce, the study we conducted, and the common features of parents' and children's experience of the separation process. They also set the stage for the later sections, which explore factors that made that process easier or harder for individual parents or children, dyads, and families.

CHAPTER 1

Changing Our Minds about Parental Divorce

If "every unhappy family is unhappy in its own way," as Tolstoy said, there is no point in looking for patterns in families' experiences of parental separation and divorce. Fortunately, after studying 160 families in which parents of school-age children separated and pursued divorces, we are convinced that Tolstoy was wrong—at least about this! We found that these unhappy families were alike in some ways and different in others. More profoundly, we found that families in which parents are divorcing are not simply unhappy; they are happy in some ways and unhappy in others. In this book, we will describe the common patterns we found and tell some of the unique stories about individuals and families we studied. What we found helped change our minds not only about what Tolstoy said, but also about the conventional view of divorce.

In this chapter we begin by reviewing some of the ways psychologists and the public think about divorce. We then introduce three of the families that participated in our project and see how their experience fits conventional wisdom. We show that current images of divorce—broken homes, dysfunctional families, selfish parents, and sad, neglected kids—do not adequately capture these three families nor the rest of the families we studied. Moreover, the experiences we learned about suggest some very different images: images of painful personal growth, increased freedom from gender-role constraints, and family reorganization and change.

This chapter was drafted by Abigail J. Stewart.

3

THINKING ABOUT PARENTAL SEPARATION
AND DIVORCE

For over a decade social scientists have pointed out that half of all children in the United States will probably spend some of their childhood in a single-parent household (see, e.g., Glick, 1979; Krantz, 1988), usually a household headed by a woman (Norton & Glick, 1986). Interestingly, this is not an entirely new phenomenon. Although the social conditions that have led to these facts are specific to our time, in earlier eras about the same number of children lived in single-parent households for other reasons, most commonly widowhood (Stannard, 1979; Dornbusch & Gray, 1988).

At least since the 1960s (when the divorce rate was judged to be rising), both public discussion and scientific research have increasingly focused on the consequences for children of various kinds of postdivorce living arrangements (see, e.g., Emery, 1988, and Furstenberg & Cherlin, 1991, for summaries). Much less research has focused on the adults involved or on the changes inside the households over the course of the marital separation and divorce (see Ahrons, 1995; Dornbusch et al., 1985; Hetherington, Cox, & Cox, 1977, 1982; and Johnston, 1993, for exceptions). In this book, we will explore parental separation and divorce as it is experienced not only by the individuals involved—both parents and children—but also in the relationships in the family (parents and children, and mothers and fathers) and in the family as a unit.

IMAGES OF DIVORCE

Many images of divorce are readily available in popular consciousness. A colleague sent us a fundraising request from a nature organization; it had a pitiful-looking bird on the envelope, and the words, "You don't have to be human to know the pain of a broken home." The most common cultural images, like this one, depict lonely, neglected children, and immature, selfish parents who are indifferent to their children's suffering and willing to "break up" a happy home. Although these images no doubt apply to some families, we found few indeed in our sample. Nevertheless, in thinking about divorce, psychologists have relied on these images, translated into professional terms. In our attempts to understand divorcing families, we too have drawn particularly on five concepts that are rough equivalents to these popular conceptions: *trauma, loss, stigma, risk,* and *life stress*. We found that these five concepts do capture some features of some family members' experience. But we also found that they keep us from seeing many other aspects of the families' experience. Specifically, they keep us from noticing how parental separation can initiate positive growth for some people, how much family members are engaged in a process of family transformation (rather than individual change), and how important gender roles are in shaping individuals' experiences of both families and separation and divorce.

THREE FAMILIES' EXPERIENCES

We will begin by describing three families who participated in our study first within a few months of the separation, and then again 1 year later. We chose these families because they illustrate the range of different types of families and divorces we heard about. Throughout most of this book we will describe results in terms of patterns and scores across the sample. But we wanted here (and wherever we can, throughout the book) to give you a sense of the lives behind those patterns and scores. In telling their stories, we have protected families' privacy by using different names and altering unimportant details. After the three families are introduced, we will consider in detail how the conventional images illuminate some features of these families' accounts, but obscure others.

The Jacksons

Jane Jackson confided early in her first interview with us, "My parents were against the marriage. They could see, I think, what I now see. I wasn't mature enough to see it." Jane recalled knowing there were serious problems in her marriage about a year after her wedding, when she was pregnant with her second child:

> "I wanted to just get out of the marriage then. . . . From that point on, I was never really happy. I think that the reality of the marriage set in, that we were not suited for each other, that we had different personalities. . . . In your early 20s you have a dream, and you're going to reach this goal. And you get near 40 and things are getting worse instead of better. You realize that the dream's never ever going to come true, unless you do something about it yourself."

It was difficult for Jane to decide to give up on her marriage. After their last child's birth, Jane and her husband grew steadily less able to work out differences in religious and other personal values, or to create an acceptable sexual relationship. By the end they were also burdened by intractable financial problems.

As John put it in his account, after 8 years of increasing marital difficulties, "The catalytic straw that broke the camel's back was money." John was accumulating debt so rapidly that it seemed to Jane the children's future educations and her everyday peace of mind were in real jeopardy. From John's perspective, Jane abandoned him to solve financial problems that he couldn't address alone. By the last year, Jane said, the couple had grown completely estranged:

> "I couldn't stand him any longer . . . I don't hate him. . . . . I just thought there was no love left, and what is the sense of staying together for what other people think when I was so miserable that I hated being home with him?"

Jane and John tried very hard to work out the ending of their marriage to be as painless as possible for their children. Jane described some of their efforts:

> "We sat down as a family and we told them that we were having problems and had decided that we would separate. And we thought the best thing was that they would just stay in the home, and I would be there. They wouldn't have to change schools; there would be as little in their life to change as possible."

Jane affirmed John's role as the children's father and the importance of his involvement in decisions about their welfare as well as their everyday life. Together Jane and John also tried to work out some financial plans and arrangements—sharing the debt liability and the family assets. Although their divorce was not conflict free, many of the Jacksons' hopes for a collaborative dissolution to their marriage were realized.

The Maxwells

Mary Maxwell's marital problems did not begin early. She told us, "We've been married 12 years and I really feel as though the first 10 years were very good." Mary and Michael had moved many times in their marriage, because of Michael's work. Mary accepted the moves, though she found them painful, and devoted herself to child rearing and volunteer activities in each new town. After the last move, though, something seemed to give:

> "We'd bought a house in the middle of a little tiny town. The children were both in school. . . . And I didn't get involved in a lot of volunteer work, which has been my pattern. . . . I purposely decided to give myself time to decide what I wanted to do. . . . And I began to feel pretty horrible."

Mary started in therapy because she felt so depressed. She gradually realized that she was very angry at her husband about their most recent move and felt it was important for them to work together on their marriage. For a while they went to a therapist together. In one therapy session a couple of months later, Mary reported that Michael said:

> " 'You've got to get your act together and decide whether you want me the way I am because this is the way I was 12 years ago when you married me and this is the way I am now and this is the way I'll always be. . . . So you decide.' I gradually came to the realization that there just wasn't any way that I could stay in this marriage because he wasn't willing to work on it."

Like the Jacksons, the Maxwells made every effort to dissolve their marriage in a way that would be relatively painless for their children. They hoped to spare them too much change. Nevertheless, they sold the house they had shared, and Mary bought a condominium in a more urban, active neighborhood. Michael searched for a job in the same area, without success, and ended up moving away. Their efforts to cooperate in making plans for the children quickly ran into trouble. They ended up in court. When the judge demanded that they come to agreement, the pressure was great enough to force them to agree on temporary arrangements. Michael agreed to support Mary and the children while Mary completed her education.

At the time of the follow-up interview, a year later, things had not worked out exactly as they had agreed. Michael—now "engaged" to someone else, though the divorce had not yet been heard in court—had not seen the children for several months and was very angry in his conversations with Mary. She reported that he said to her, "I have a life of my own to lead. If you're going to do this to me, and if push comes to shove and it means going to jail, you can starve to death for all I care." During this period, Mary and Michael had been unable to come to agreement about the terms of the settlement, so the contested divorce was still tied up in the courts. Mary felt good about her improved relationship with the children, her education, her new and moderately serious relationship, and her future, but she was concerned about the fact that the children were not seeing their father very much. The children themselves mentioned missing him and wishing they could see him more. Even so, 10-year-old Maureen said, "I don't really care [about my parents being divorced] because they were always fighting when they were together. It doesn't bother me, other than missing my father." She also said that at this point (18 months after the separation) "they're not yelling. In the beginning, when they first got separated, Mommy was always angry. She took it out on us—she'd yell at us and get uptight. Now she doesn't do it anymore."

Clearly the Maxwells went through more conflict than did the Jacksons.

Yet their experiences were similar in one basic respect: Both families transformed their no-longer-satisfactory family situation into one in which the mother and children formed one household and the father (first alone, eventually with others) formed another. Though this is a common pattern, it is by no means universal, as we can see in the next family.

The Andersons

The Anderson family's transformation took a different form. Although Art was unemployed at the time of the separation, the children stayed with him because Alice simply left one day and called to say she wouldn't be back. She had been in and out of treatment for substance abuse for some time. Art told us:

> "She saw the program didn't work. Things weren't getting better at home. She was still arguing with the kids all the time, and she was generally miserable. I don't know if the [substance problem] would have reached the heights it did if it wasn't for the business failure. I think that had a lot to do with it."

Before Alice left, the family had many problems. Art felt Alice was a very poor parent. As he put it:

> "A good parent is in my eyes someone that sees to your every need when you need them. That's when you're very young—from infancy to 7 or 8, and then to a lesser degree after that, and as they become teenagers to a lesser degree. Parenting changes as they get older. But she was a parent that characteristically never prepared breakfast for her children, no matter what age they were; prepared very poor meals, if meals at all."

One child, Alexander, was having serious difficulties. According to Art:

> "[Alice] would get home from work early, and she would proceed to get bombed. And she'd be pretty much gone by 5 o'clock. And there'd be confrontations with Alexander. My daughter didn't stay around for them as much as Alexander did. She'd disappear and go in her room when the arguments would come. Alexander would stay around and argue back, which didn't do him any good. So our nights were like, I'd be trying to act as a mediator, trying to tune her out as much as I could so she wouldn't affect me that much. Whenever the confrontation got heated enough, then I would jump into it, break it up."

After the separation, Art said:

> "Things are easier. It's different. The house is a lot quieter than it was. It's more calm. I think the kids will agree that, even though Alexander's still himself, it's more calm. I don't believe that the kids have any desire to see things return to the way they were—and I certainly don't."

Like many custodial mothers, Art felt that he was the custodial parent by default. Although he felt that the household was more of a responsibility after the separation, it was also more pleasant.

COMPARING IMAGES AND EXPERIENCES

Do These Separations Seem "Traumatic"?

The notion of trauma assumes that divorce is an "event" occurring in an otherwise benign stream of events, which leaves painful consequences in its wake (see Hetherington, 1979, for a similar critique). The popular understanding of "trauma" is quite consistent with that of psychologists; that is, a catastrophic event occurs suddenly and leaves lasting and serious scars. The Andersons' divorce has some of the hallmarks of trauma. For example, it was sudden. Alice Anderson simply left one day, and the rest of the family had to cope with the resulting feelings. Eighteen months after her mother left, Anita (the daughter) said that she could not understand divorce, because "if I care about someone, no matter how bad something happens, I'm not just going to walk away from them, because there must be a problem there and they're going to need someone." Interestingly, though, Anita went on to make clear that the puzzle she was trying to solve was not why or how her mother could leave her, but how her *father* could have failed her mother so. As she put it:

> "That's something that I resent my father for—because there was a time when my mother was having problems and he, sort of, not physically deserted her, but mentally cut himself away from her and that's not right. You should make it work at all costs, if you really care about that person."

Anita's feelings about her situation were very complicated. She said that she was glad that her mother left and that it was "quieter" without her. She described herself as having been "helped" by her mother leaving, but she also missed her and found it hard to be the only female in the household. Although Anita's feelings about her family situation were too complex to summarize as only reflecting "trauma," she suspected that her brother, Alexander, had a less ambivalent response to his mother's departure. She felt that "he's very bitter about the whole thing" and "suffered a lot because of what happened."

However, Alexander himself said the divorce "doesn't really matter much. It actually helps a little. Because I'm doing a little better in school. Since my mother's not there." He also indicated that *he* thought *Anita* was more bothered than he was about the divorce. Alexander's advice to children whose parents were divorcing was "Well, take it easy. Don't think it's the end of the world. Thinking about it won't make it better, and . . . worrying about it isn't going to help the situation."

Alexander had been viewed as having problems before the separation and had been given special treatment. He continued to have problems at school at about the same level after the separation. Thus, although the concept of "trauma" may help us understand some aspects of Alexander's experience, it ignores his persistent real problems, which began long before the separation, as well as his own conscious view that the separation was "not the end of the world." It also requires us to ignore Alice Anderson's substance problem and the possibility that she simply could not solve it within this family. As Anita said in the second-year interview, "Well, she's getting help now and she wouldn't go and try to get help when she was with us, but when she left she did. She went into a hospital." Before the separation Alice's behavior was clearly a painful feature of the Anderson family's daily life; it seems clear that Alice's departure alleviated that pain for her and the others—an outcome hard to recognize under the rubric of trauma.

It is even more difficult to think of the Jacksons' divorce as involving "trauma" for their children. All the children seemed to adjust well in the aftermath of the parental separation. Clearly Jane was much happier in that period, too. It could be argued that John Jackson had real difficulty recovering from the separation; in the second interview he said, "I think the arrangement right now stinks." He was angry about the financial settlement, angry that he felt shut out of his children's lives, and frustrated by continuing business difficulties. These responses, though unhappy, do not fit the definition of "trauma" at all well.

The Maxwells' divorce involved careful planning and preparation, as well as family therapy for the new single-parent household. Although everyone in the family had some low points and difficulties, they were relieved by the reduction in tension, and Mary developed new strengths and plans. Eighteen months after the separation she said, "I have been feeling really strong and really healthy, and I've begun to enjoy life again." Although we had no direct contact with Michael, we cannot describe anyone we did see in the Maxwell family as traumatized by the divorce.

The image of trauma, then, has only limited application to the families described here. Why should this image be such a powerful, readily available one? We suspect that the notion that divorce is traumatic arises in part from a desire to distance ourselves from divorce, to see it as equivalent to rare and terrible events, rather than as frequent and the result of gradually accumulating tensions. An additional factor may be a tendency to think about divorce in clinical terms, that is, from the perspective of clients or patients who feel unable to cope with painful events in their past (Wallerstein & Kelly, 1980; Wallerstein & Blakeslee, 1989). When a divorce involves the sudden, irreversible abandonment of a child (or sometimes an adult), it may indeed be traumatic, particularly if that abandonment is difficult to explain or overcome. But in the three families we have examined, as in our study as a whole, the notion of trauma is inconsistent with the more typical pattern: a long period of unhappiness and struggle that preceded the separation, children suffering obvious pain in the presence of unhappy parents still living together but in conflict, and most family members adapting to their new situation relatively quickly.

Do Parental Separation and Divorce Produce Painful Losses?

The notion of "loss," with attendant concepts of grief and mourning, has been stressed by those particularly concerned about the fact that divorce involves the departure, or absence, of one of the parents from the child-rearing household. After one parent leaves a household, children usually feel sad and wish they could see that parent more; this aspect of children's experience is highlighted by a focus on loss. Members of all three of the families described some "losses" that came with the divorce. To focus on those exclusively, though, obscures the gains they also reported.

For example, Mark Maxwell reported feeling "fine" about the divorce in both interviews; he also said that he wished he saw his father more. Maureen, his older sister, felt "a little" sad after the separation, but was also relieved about it. Jimmy Jackson said he was sad and upset when his parents told him about the divorce, and during the first-year interview he said that if a magician could give him three wishes, his first would be for his parents to get back together. However, by the second-year interview he said, "It's almost the same as when they were married, 'cause I see my mother a lot and my father a lot."

Some parents clearly felt their losses consciously, even when they had sought the divorce. Mary Maxwell, 18 months after the separation, advised that those who are divorcing should

"do the best you can to save it [your marriage], but when you get to the point where there's just no saving it, feel good about having made the decision. But then go on to . . . kind of give yourself at least a year of mourning, because it's ... you know, I can't imagine anything more painful, unless maybe it would be the death of a child or someone very close to me."

In contrast to these complex responses, the Andersons' separation was apparently a relief to everyone right away. Art reported that even Alexander was "relieved; he was happy. I think he probably would have preferred that it had happened even sooner." By the second interview Art continued to feel that "not having her around the house is definitely a plus," but he also said that "I don't have much of a life; it's an existence is all. . . . Having the whole load is the hardest thing." Art's daughter, Anita, was aware of the gains rather than the losses in her family situation; in the first interview she said that "it's better every way around" and "it's a lot more normal." She pointed out, "I've never really had a nuclear family, 'cause my mother's never been there. They [other kids] think it's terrible. I don't think so 'cause I've been living with it since I was little."

Of course there *were* losses in the course of this parental divorce, and it would be wrong to overlook them. By the second year Anita said of her mother, "I miss her sometimes because it's hard living in a house with all boys. Sometimes I wish she were there, and then, when she is, I just go crazy." Anita felt that their mother's absence had wounded Alexander more. She said, "I was helped by the fact that she left but he suffered from it by not having her around." It is testimony to the power of the *concept* of parental divorce as loss that Anita attributes Alexander's problems to his mother's absence despite her clear recognition (and her father's) that Alexander's behavior problems *decreased* after his mother's departure. Finally, Alexander himself reported that although his sister told him she'd developed stomachaches because of the divorce, his father "seems a lot more relieved." He also said, "I see [my mother] the right amount," and she "seems real happy. I figure that means she's got a load off her mind."

The notion of loss clearly does capture some important features of the experience of divorce and separation for both children and parents. Children miss their absent parents, and parents grieve for the loss of their earlier dreams, as well as for a particular family life now definitively closed to them. Thinking about divorce exclusively as loss makes it difficult to see and understand the anger experienced about a past that was disappointing and infuriating, the relief experienced as strains end, and the optimism and hope resulting from the sense of new possibilities opening up. In addition, perhaps the most important problem with a focus on loss is the way in which it keeps attention on the past rather than the present and future. Divorcing parents and their children are in current relationships with each other and are observing each other in the present. They are not only, or perhaps even mainly, working through a past set of relationships; they are working out new and future ones.

Do Parents and Children Feel Stigmatized by Divorce?

Divorcing parents and their children also must work out new relationships with the rest of their social network—extended family, neighbors, friends, schoolmates, teachers, and coworkers. In the past it has been suggested that divorce is a negatively sanctioned family change, one that carries with it a burden of stigma. Divorces are often thought of as marriages that "failed," families in which a divorce has occurred are often described as "broken homes" (see Thornton, 1989), and the offspring in these families are labeled "children of divorce," as if the divorce defined their very nature (see, e.g., Guttmann, Geva, & Gefen, 1988). On the other hand, as divorce has become more common, it has been generally assumed that the stigma associated with parental divorce has lessened, both for adults and for children. While there may indeed be an average reduction in the experience of stigma associated with divorce, it is also true that the divorcing families in our sample ranged widely in the degree to which their family situation felt like a social burden, or stigma.

For Jane Jackson, anxiety about "disgracing the families" was a factor that kept her in the marriage. She and her husband both came from families in which there had "never ever been a separation." Some of Jane's social discomfort was clearly related to her "single" status; she felt observed and judged during the early postseparation period. In that first stage, Jane said:

> "Right now I'd just like to start a life of my own again. To be free to do what I want to do without living in a suburban neighborhood where everyone sort of watches you—'Aha, she's going out tonight. Aha, she's doing this or that.' I just want to get over that."

Jane felt that what she was going through was private, and she was uncomfortable about being the object of gossip:

> "I would not advertise it. I feel that it's a very personal and intimate experience, and I feel that it's only those affected by my separation that need to be privy to it. Otherwise I feel it's just idle gossip that goes in one ear and out the other. And people love to hear what has happened to you."

By the follow-up interview, Jane was more philosophical about the issue of gossip, but her new perspective on the whole period made it clear that she continued to feel that her divorce was a social liability. In response to a question about what had been surprising about the process of separation and divorce, she said:

> "Well, one thing has—people's attitudes. In the beginning you are a subject of gossip, rumors, whatever you want to call it. 'Oh, how terri-

ble,' you know . . . 'How could she do that to him?' 'How could he do that to her?' Then you come full circle, and I hear more people say, 'I'm so glad they got divorced; I could never see them together anymore.' People that in the beginning didn't want to get involved; all of a sudden, people aren't afraid of you anymore . . . they see that you are a mother first, and you are not a barfly. You know, I'm very much a homebody, and I'm not going to disgrace the neighborhood and disgrace the children. I think time takes care of an awful lot of things. I was very caught up in the beginning with what people thought. Being the first divorce in the neighborhood, I just thought I disgraced everyone. And then I finally said, you know, nobody has to live my life but me, and what do I care what anyone thinks? Why it happened—it's nobody's business."

To some degree, Jane's feelings about the separation colored her son's experience. Jimmy reported that he knew other kids whose parents were separated, but he didn't talk to them about his parents' separation because "my mother told me not to; she doesn't want anyone to know." However, by the follow-up interview he indicated that he did talk to other children with separated parents about his own family situation. Even in the early period, his sisters, Josie and Julie, were talking to their friends about their parents' situation. Later Josie mentioned that she also talked with friends whose parents were not separated or divorced, because they were curious about the experience. Clearly the children did not feel as self-conscious about their family situation as Jane did.

For Jane Jackson, the experience of separation and divorce involved transition from a social status in which she felt valued and acceptable (wife) to one in which she felt like an outcast (divorcée, potential "barfly," disgrace). Over time, she was relieved to discover that the status of "mother," and her personal characteristics, seemed to compensate for her lowered, and risky, social position. John Jackson, though embedded in a very similar social network, did not report these kinds of concerns. During the follow-up interview, 18 months after the separation, he was somewhat troubled about the problem—as a devout Catholic—of remarriage. He did not, though, seem to have any sense of social disgrace about the divorce, perhaps because he did not seek it, or perhaps because—at least in some circles—divorcing men are less vulnerable to being judged immoral than are divorcing women.

No one in the Maxwell family reported any stigma surrounding the separation and divorce. Mary mentioned that

"I'm somewhat of an oddity, and people are . . . I feel as though I know a lot of people who care about me. I suppose they're somewhat curious, too, not having gone through this kind of thing themselves. And there are people who I see at church that I only see once a week, but they're interested and seem to be caring."

No doubt because of her sense of her friends and neighbors as curious and caring, rather than critical or judgmental, Mary found it easy to talk to people about the separation. She said, "I'm pretty open about talking about it, because I have found in the past that it's not good not to talk about the things that are affecting you drastically."

None of the Anderson family focused on the separation and divorce as a source of social discomfort, in part because the family had so many other problems. Art mentioned that he thought Anita was helped by talking with other kids about her various problems at home:

> "She's finding out she's not so unique. There are several of her fellow students having the same or worse problems at home. So she, I'm sure, thought that she was the only person in the world suffering this. Now she's finding out that she's got a lot of girlfriends that have the same problem."

In fact, Anita did report that she talked a lot with her friends, and that "just about all of them" had divorced parents: "We all hang together because we all have the same problems." Nevertheless, Anita did report some discomfort with her extended family. She mentioned that one household

> "invited us to a Christmas party, and I felt kind of out of place, but they made me feel welcome. It's my mother who was out of place there. They'll take in my father and me and my mother doesn't fit in, because they look at her as 'You left, and you deserted the whole clan.' I feel sorry for her; I don't see that that's her fault."

It does seem, then, that Anita felt that her mother was judged by some for leaving the household; she had a sense of her mother being "stigmatized," but more than that Anita reported a powerful sense that her family had never been "normal." Any stigma associated with the divorce was minor compared with her sense that her home life had always been painful and inadequate.

Does Divorce Put Children "At Risk" for Other Problems in the Future?

Partly because of the association of parental divorce with notions of trauma, loss, and stigma, divorce is often assumed to increase children's risk of psychopathology and/or inadequate adult relationships (see Kulka & Wein-garten, 1979). Adults experiencing separation and divorce are, in this perspective, also considered "at risk" because of the association between stress and psychopathology. Although evaluating these kinds of outcomes requires a fairly long timespan for full assessment, we were able to explore the relatively short-term (18-month) impact of parental separation and divorce on the various family members, in their own and each other's eyes.

Three major themes emerged from reviewing the experience of the three families described in this chapter:

1. Parents (and children, to a lesser extent) were very concerned about the possibility that the separation and divorce would create long-term problems for the children.
2. Many observed that the separation brought about an improvement in day-to-day life, and therefore in "mental health."
3. Other aspects of the family's history—for example, many moves for the Maxwells, substance abuse and family disorganization for the Andersons, and long-term behavior problems for Alexander Anderson—were generally more important factors than divorce in family members' problems.

Perhaps because the Maxwell family's separation did not seem well defined as trauma, loss, or stigma, no family members seemed particularly concerned about each others' responses to the divorce as putting them "at risk." In discussing her children's adjustment to the family situation, Mary said:

"Let me point this out. Mike always traveled, so I was the one with the kids nearly every week. In terms of separation, it wasn't any big deal there. You know, after he had been gone about 3 or 4 months, I said to the kids, 'How do you feel about Dad being gone?' They both agreed that it was just like his being on a business trip, only this time it was longer."

Moreover, after the separation Mary and the children stopped moving so often. They had moved 14 times in the preceding 10 years, but had now lived in one town for almost 4 years—the longest they ever had stayed in one place. Mary felt the difficult aspect of the separation for her children was her own emotional life:

"I lost my temper very quickly and I spent a lot of time feeling real sad. But I tried to be open about that and show them how I was feeling. . . . Probably it was hard for them at times to see me feeling so angry or feeling so sad a lot of the time."

In the long run, though, Mary felt that the "kids are doing fine. I'm not real concerned. I feel like I'm doing the best things that I can to help them." In short, continuing the marriage would have presented more problems for the children, and the separation actually lowered the children's "risk" of difficulties by lowering the tension in their lives.

Everyone in the Jackson family reported that after the separation Jimmy Jackson's behavior improved dramatically. Jane said:

> "Jimmy was completely out of control temper-wise when his father was there and it was growing worse and worse by the year. When his father was gone about 3 weeks, it stopped. There was an abrupt change, and as each week went on I could see that . . . his temper tantrums were getting less and less"

A year later, Jane confirmed this account, reporting that "within a few weeks of my husband and I separating, all of this behavior stopped." Even John Jackson felt there was no doubt that Jimmy's behavior was radically improved after the separation, and he said, "I am not afraid to say that very possibly my leaving the house is responsible for him doing better. . . . If it is, then I'm glad I left."

Finally, the Anderson family—which had struggled with so many problems over time—seemed generally to agree that the separation and divorce had reduced the overall strain in the household, and thereby, if anything, had lowered everyone's risk.

Is Parental Separation and Divorce a "Life Stress" That Demands Coping from Family Members?

The risk associated with divorce needs to be contextualized in terms of the entire family history. The life stress it generates must also be considered in that context. By linking parental divorce with other life stresses, researchers emphasize the potential for coping, though this often introduces a troubling tendency to divide those who experience divorce into successful copers versus failures, ignoring the complexities of most people's continuing, always only partially successful, efforts. It is clear, though, that parental divorce can introduce new stresses into family members' lives and can demand new coping efforts. For the Andersons, interestingly, although many stresses ended with the separation (fights and scenes), many financial problems continued. There were also some new stresses—particularly for Anita. As she pointed out, "I got left with the responsibility of the house." On the other hand, by the time of the follow-up, Anita had given up trying to run the household and did not try to prepare meals. At that time, her father reported that "having the whole load is the hardest thing." The period after the separation certainly demanded "coping" efforts from Alice and from Art, but the period before the separation had been demanding too. On the whole, both Alice and Art felt that the stress level was lower after the separation.

For different reasons, the same was true for the Maxwells. Although Mary felt there was a period shortly after the separation when her emotional life produced some stress for her children, by the time of the follow-up she described Mark as "more carefree. He seems to have more fun, and feel better about being away from me and playing with friends." The one later stress that anyone mentioned was the parents' telephone interactions. Maureen said, "I haven't heard one time when they have hung up without fighting." However, the major release associated with the divorce was the ending of the parents' fighting in the household. As Maureen mentioned in the same interview, in the past

"we could hear them all the way across the street. Like one time we were outside, we were out in the back, and we were playing on the swing set. . . . And they were yelling—I mean, my friend up the road heard it. She came down, she goes, 'What's going on here?' I go, 'Shhh, they're having a fight.' . . . And you could hear every word they said."

For the Jackson family, there were some definite life stresses associated with the separation. In the early period, Jane Jackson reported that she found the "sense of responsibility" stressful:

"I'm far more hectic. It isn't more hectic in the house; it's much calmer in the house. The atmosphere is much more tranquil in the house, but, inside of me, I am constantly on the go."

Jane also felt that the children found their new financial situation stressful:

"I have never said anything against him as such, but when it got to, 'Why can't I have this? Why can't I have that?' I felt that the children had to know that I wasn't receiving any support. . . . I just felt that I could not take the brunt of their anger about why they couldn't have things when it was not my fault. I was doing as much as I could."

Finally, in the early period there was stress associated with John Jackson's visits with his children. Jane felt that Jimmy was "very high-strung after being with his father. He returns to what he was before." However, a year later, when John was visiting much less often, Jane felt that, for Jimmy, "his father's seeming rejection must be very hard for him. . . . I'm sure he looks around and sees his friends with their fathers . . . and their fathers are faithful in taking them . . . and I think this bothers him." John himself reported that he felt the visits were now "strained" and that the kids seemed "uncomfortable" with him.

Despite the tension over the visits, Jane felt at the follow-up that a great deal of discord was now "out of the way." The children were also comfortable with the household situation; in fact, Julie reported that her mother could now "handle everything better—like she's more organized with bills." Focusing on individual stresses, and individuals' coping efforts, tends to ignore positive changes and the overall texture of daily life, as well as aspects of people's experience—including their feelings and understandings—that do not call for active coping.

NEW IMAGES OF DIVORCE

We have seen that the conventional images of divorce obscure some important features of family members' experience. Three new images capture important aspects of our families' experiences that are ignored or glossed over by the conventional images: divorce as an opportunity for change and growth, divorce as a family transformation, and divorce as changing the pattern of gender roles in a family.

Can Divorce, Like Other Life Changes, Provide an Opportunity for Growth?

Individual members of all three families could identify positive changes in their individual lives that were a function of the family change. For example, Mary Maxwell thought that Mark had a better social life because she and the children had moved to a less isolated neighborhood after the separation. Mary's own social life also changed:

> "Mike and I were really kind of limited to—consciously or maybe unconsciously, I don't know—limited to people very similar to us: other couples with young children. I'm sure that becoming involved in feminist issues and things of that kind led me to seek different ways of having friends, in terms of having women friends that were not necessarily married, or not necessarily married to people that Mark would want to know."

Overall, Mary felt that "I'm improving all the time" and that the divorce had "changed everything":

> "It's changed my expectations of what I can and will accomplish. There have been so many ways . . . that it showed me that I can get through

something like this . . . and I can benefit from it in some ways. A lot of times I feel very free and very excited about a life of my own."

John Jackson felt his divorce had led to changes in his social network and his relationships with other people. He said the separation "has made me have a much better self-image . . . because . . . almost immediately there was the outpouring of help from friends—people who weren't family." John also felt he had created new and deeper relationships in his life. In particular, he and his brother had grown very close since the separation.

The Anderson family members mostly did not report personal growth or change as a result of the separation. But both children suspected that their mother had in fact benefited from it in just this way. Alexander said his mother had "changed a lot" in that "she's gotten a lot healthier" since the separation. Anita felt that her mother was now willing to seek help for her problems, and that "she's an independent person, and she's glad that she's not tied down." Anita elaborated, "She's more optimistic than she was. She has a purpose. She wants to come back in the spring; she wants to get a job, and she started running and everything."

In fact, all of the adults we talked with felt they had (and were perceived by their children as having) grown and developed as a result of the separation. The three women were all viewed—by themselves or others—as having increased self-confidence and self-direction; in Mary Maxwell's case, this included making some new kinds of friends. Separation and divorce may provide adults more than children with special opportunities for growth, but there may also be growth-promoting aspects of divorce for children too. In particular, as we will see in Chapter 4, it may enhance children's capacity to empathize with other people, and may increase their independence and self-reliance. Focusing on the opportunities for growth does help bring positive changes into view, but we are still only considering the individual family member, rather than the family as an integrated unit.

Does Parental Divorce Produce a Transformation of the Family, Rather than a "Broken Home"?

When researchers' focus has widened from individuals to the household, they have found that the household and family as a unit is transformed by parental separation (Ahrons & Wallisch, 1987; Camara & Resnick, 1987, 1989; Hetherington, 1987; Hetherington & Arasteh, 1988; Hetherington et al., 1977; Vincent, 1987). That is, it is not merely that an individual leaves, and other individuals respond to that departure, but that the family system changes in complex ways as a result of the separation. We have already commented on some of those changes—changes in the atmosphere or level of tension in the household, in the amount of conflict or fighting, and in the level of disorganization. Other changes were observed as well.

Mary Maxwell mentioned that in the beginning she missed her husband's help with the evening routines, and that therefore "I think I would like to try getting [the children] involved in chores of this kind." By the second interview, the evening routines had indeed changed:

> "Mark likes to help me in the kitchen; Maureen's not real big on that, although I do make her do it sometimes. I just feel that they should both help out in the kitchen somewhat. Mark really enjoys it, and certain things Maureen likes too."

This kind of organization of children into collective household maintenance activities was a common solution to the problem of needing simultaneously to get the work done, pay attention to children's conversation, and provide companionship.

Anita Anderson felt that her household had changed dramatically, but not so much in terms of the routines. She noticed the change in family dynamics. She said:

> "I'm glad that [my mother]'s gone now because there was so much going on in the house: My mother not getting along with my father; my brother aggravating my mother; my mother taking that out on me. And me just walking away, and then me getting in trouble for walking away when she was talking to me. So it's a lot better."

One family dynamic that seemed strengthened by the separation in all three families was the children's awareness of their ability to rely on each other. Anita commented that she thought it was easier if you have a sibling when your parents get divorced because "you've got someone else to rely on other than just the other parent." Alexander independently commented that "we both knew about what was going on, so we could both talk about the same thing." Even more strikingly, Maureen Maxwell indicated that she "made a difference" to Mark, "probably for support and stuff—like, if he said, 'Mommy is being mean to me,' he'd come over to me." Jimmy Jackson also commented that "if I had any question they [his sisters] would answer it." One sister also mentioned the presence of her siblings was helpful, because without them "the mother would be working and you'd have no one to talk to and just be sitting home alone." The other agreed that "if there was something to joke about, you weren't left by yourself to think. You could always get your mind off it by talking to them or something." However, she felt that she and her siblings did not talk about the separation directly because "none of us want to really talk about it to anyone in the family because they might feel differently and then you'd get into a fight or something."

Looking exclusively at individual change after parental separations and divorces makes it difficult to see the ways in which families are changing as a whole. One difference when families change is the way in which gender is experienced in the family.

How Does Gender Complicate the Experience of Parental Separation and Divorce?

Although the question of sex differences in children's reactions to parental divorce has been examined extensively (see Zaslow, 1988, 1989, for reviews), the process of separation and divorce has generally been viewed as the same experience for all adults, male and female (see Riessman, 1990, and Ahrons, 1995, for important exceptions). When differences have been observed, they have usually been limited to postdivorce adjustment and financial difficulties, and have been attributed to postseparation custody arrangements, men's greater earning power, or greater male vulnerability to relational losses. Increasingly, though, it has been suggested that because marital and parental roles are themselves gendered (see, e.g., Thompson & Walker, 1989), perhaps the *experience* of divorce (rather than the amount of pain) is systematically different for adult men and women (Allen, 1993; Kurz, 1995; Rice, 1994). It may also be that children experience their own roles in their families in gendered terms; if so, parental divorce and the postseparation household may be "gendered" as well.

We have already pointed to some of the differences in women's and men's experiences of personal growth following the separation; these differences may in fact derive from differences in the preseparation households. As Mary Maxwell said, "In a lot of ways I've been a pretty traditional homemaker and a mother. I've been at home with the children, and I've done a lot of volunteer work." Moreover, Mary's husband (as mentioned earlier) viewed their separation as a result of her desire for greater independence than the marriage had provided. Mary's interest in feminism—which, after all, offers an explicit analysis of gender relations—might be one source of their emphasis on the gendered features of their family life.

However, the Jacksons' family life was also explicitly discussed in gender terms. John Jackson believed that his wife was disappointed in his performance of a heterosexual masculine role. In support of this view, he quoted his wife as saying, "Don't cross your legs like that—you look like a fairy." He also said, "I'm a very emotional person. I'm very close to the surface, and I don't consider it unmanly to cry. She does."

In fact, Jane Jackson cited "lack of respect" as the reason for the divorce and indicated that she felt "he had a childish image of what love was—pleasing the mother, doing things to please—rather than an adult relationship of give and take." Although she did not describe him as insufficiently "masculine," she did describe him as immature, and the two concepts may have been close to opposite in her mind or his.

The Anderson household after the separation felt extremely gendered to Anita. She felt her father wasn't interested in the same kinds of things she was:

> "He's the basic jock type; he wants Alexander to do what Alexander wants to do, and if I'm not doing sports I have to do sports. It really kills me because I'm, like, 'Dad, I'm not a jock. Leave me alone.' And if I'm not doing that—I'm not a boy, so there's nothing he can relate to 'cause that's what he is."

As we noted earlier, Anita felt that despite the problems living with her mother, "it's hard living in a house with all boys." In addition, Anita was concerned about the consequences of the divorce for Alexander's relations with women: "Alexander doesn't understand both sides; he understands my father's side." She pointed out that

> "he doesn't relate to females at all. We just got a form from school saying that he can talk to males. He has all these counselors and will talk to the guy but he won't talk to the girl . . . he's just not very open to women."

In all three families, then, gender was an explicit part of individuals' understanding of their family lives, sometimes before and sometimes after the separation. In addition, other aspects of family lives—such as differential access to economic and other resources—are rooted in cultural gender norms and structures, but are usually not part of the family members' conscious thinking about gender and their families.

OUR WAY OF LOOKING AT PARENTAL
SEPARATION AND DIVORCE

In our view, all of the images examined in this chapter demonstrated some utility in thinking about parental separation and divorce. As we've seen, the images most closely tied to a clinical perspective (trauma, loss, stigma, risk, life stress) also share a number of liabilities for understanding the phenomena associated with divorce in the general population. First, these images often treat parental separation and divorce as a single event with consequences, rather than as one event in a complex family history. Second, they tend to exclude from view any possible positive aspects of the experience. Finally, they keep our focus exclusively on the individual level.

Our perspective on parental separation and divorce attempts to include attention to those aspects of the experience that are indeed well described as trauma, loss, stigma, risk, and life stress, but to include other critical features as well. Thus, we see parental separation and divorce as a process of family transformation that both results from and produces individual and family changes—some of which are losses or traumatic, and some of which are beneficial. Moreover, we see the very concept of "family" as containing powerful associations with gender, including normative definitions of fathers, mothers, daughters, and sons.

In the next chapter we will examine the connections between the kinds of questions researchers want to answer—often framed in terms of the concepts outlined in this chapter—and their research designs. We will also describe our study, and the kinds of questions our design allowed us to address.

CHAPTER 2

Studying Family Transformation
RESEARCH DESIGNS AND THE FAMILY CHANGES PROJECT

We have seen in Chapter 1 how images of divorce can both reveal and conceal different aspects of people's experience. It is clear that the way we think about divorce affects what we learn from families we study. It also affects the research design we use, and every decision we make about the research design increases our chances of seeing some things and missing others. The critical task for the researcher, then, is not to design the "perfect" study (perfect for what?), but to understand and take account of the things any given study can reveal, as well as what it may leave obscure. In our case we needed a design that allowed us to document the course of people's experience of the early stages of parental separation and divorce and to examine factors that made that experience more or less difficult.

HOW DO RESEARCHERS STUDY DIVORCE?

Researchers have used four major research designs to study the psychological meaning of parental divorce: control group, multiple comparison groups, comparative divorce groups, and within-group longitudinal. These designs have most often been used to study divorce in terms of the popular images of divorce discussed in the last chapter (see Table 2.1 for a summary of their

This chapter was drafted by Abigail J. Stewart.

TABLE 2.1. Four Research Designs for Studying Divorce

Design	Advantages	Questions
Control group design		
Compare families with divorce to families without	Can identify differences between families where there is a divorce versus not	(1) Can we believe the two kinds of families only differ in one way—divorce? (2) Are divorcing families all similar, and different from all "intact" families? (3) Will the "intact" families never have a divorce? Are the ones that will divorce different from the ones that will not? (4) Does time since divorce matter?
Multiple comparison groups design		
Compare divorcing families to at least two kinds of "intact" families, for example, high conflict, no divorce versus low conflict, no divorce versus divorce	Can differentiate among families where there is no divorce and identify differences between families where there is a divorce versus each of the other groups	(1) Are the critical differences captured by these groups? (2), (3), and (4): Same as above.
Comparative divorce groups design		
Compare different divorce situations, for example, mother versus father custody	Can examine role of a particular difference between divorcing families	(1) Are the critical differences captured by these groups? (2) Is this dimension of divorce the only or most important one? (3) and (4): Same as above.
Within-group longitudinal design		
Compare divorcing families to each other and over time	No assumptions about what is most important aspect of divorce; permits comparison of divorcing families to each other along many dimensions, and over time	Cannot attribute findings to divorce per se

strengths and weaknesses). In this chapter we will describe the four designs, because they appear so commonly in discussions of research on divorce. We will explain why one of these designs suited our purposes and describe the choices we made. Then we will describe our project in detail.

The Control Group Design

Judging from public and professional responses to most studies of the consequences of parental divorce, the research design assumed to be most valuable involves direct comparison of families (or family members) in which there has been a divorce and families in which there has not. If a researcher's focus is on the potential of parental divorce to produce trauma, loss, and psychological risk, naturally it makes good sense to compare individuals who have and have not experienced the relevant "risk factor." Substantively, studies comparing "intact" families and divorcing families usually address the psychological adjustment of individuals in and (to a lesser degree) the adequacy of the functioning of the postdivorce family. The control group design promises identification of amounts of damage to the specific domains of individual and family adjustment after parental divorce. Such information is clearly of urgent importance to those interested in policy and intervention strategies to support and help those "hurt" by parental divorce.

However, the control group design also depends on a number of assumptions about parental divorce. First, and most crucially, it assumes that it is possible to identify two groups of families that differ only in terms of the presence or absence of a divorce. If the researcher cannot successfully identify two groups that differ *only* in terms of divorce, how can we attribute differences between the two groups to parental divorce? If the two groups of families differ in other ways (e.g., if there is more violence, economic instability, personal psychopathology, or family disorganization in one group than the other), then any differences between them in postdivorce adjustment could be a function of these other differences. Generally, the control group design assumes that the differences *among* families in which there has been a divorce and *among* families in which there has not are trivial, relative to the difference divorce itself makes. We question that assumption.

More problematically, comparative studies must assume that families in which there will never be a divorce are equivalent to families in which there has not yet been a divorce, but will be; thus, the identification of "intactness" (or nondivorce) at one moment in time is sufficient. Although there is little longitudinal research directly assessing the plausibility of this assumption, Block, Block, and Gjerde (1986) found that children of couples who divorced by the time their children were 14 already differed at age 3 (and at every age in between) from the children whose parents remained married (at least until their children were 14). This finding suggests that the households of families where there is eventually a divorce may indeed differ from those in which there is never one, in ways that are quite relevant to child adjustment.

Similarly, studies employing a control group design often assume that the effects of divorce are uniform not only across families, but also over time; thus, the effects of divorce are permanent and unchanging. As a result of this assumption, it is possible to treat as equivalent the impact of parental divorces that took place only a few months before and those of many years ago.

If any of these assumptions is implausible, a design in which families where there has been a divorce are compared with those where there has not runs the risks of misattributing discovered differences to divorce and of not finding out about important differences among families. Particular studies comparing families in which there has been a divorce with those in which there hasn't can avoid some of these assumptions and thereby some of these risks. For example, a researcher can focus on the short-term impact of divorce (thus assuming that time since divorce does matter) and can attempt to assess some of the likeliest differences between families with and without divorces that might be alternative explanations of different adjustment outcomes. Comparisons between families with and without divorce experience can "control for" predivorce violence and conflict, economic instability, psychopathology, and/or family disorganization, either by taking those variables into account when selecting families for inclusion in the study, or by assessing these variables and introducing them as statistical controls in analyses.

Use of control strategies certainly increases our confidence in the attribution of effects to parental divorce, though one can never be certain that all potential confounding differences between the two groups have been assessed. If, however, we have serious questions about the uniformity of the experience of parental divorce—and the experience of marital "intactness"!— and we are interested in exploring the variations among families in which there has or has not been a divorce, then improving or strengthening these designs may not satisfy us. It is important to stress, though, that this latter issue is an issue of interest and not one of absolute "value." Studies comparing families with and without divorce—if they attend to the problematic or unjustified assumptions a simple comparison might suggest—are useful in producing one important kind of knowledge: assessment of the degree and domain of compromise or adjustment attributable to parental divorce. This is not, however, the only possible interesting question about parental divorce.

The Multiple Comparison Groups Design

A second, fairly common research design for studying the impact of parental divorce involves comparison of families in which there has been a divorce (with and without high predivorce conflict), families in which there is high parental conflict but no divorce, and families in which there is low conflict and no divorce. This comparison is a most useful one for addressing the question of whether it is divorce per se that is the critical event compromising children's adjustment (as, e.g., the trauma, loss, and risk concepts would suggest) or whether parental conflict might be the critical factor that is associated with, but not the same as, divorce (as, e.g., the stress and family system concepts might suggest). This design, then, introduces parental conflict as a potential alternative source of adjustment difficulties, and thus highlights one presumed feature differentiating families in which there has been and those in which there has not been a parental divorce. In terms of children's current adjustment difficulties, research using this second type of design has produced valuable information about the relative equivalence of parental divorce and parental conflict without divorce. Nevertheless, the other assumptions associated with the first comparative design hold for all other kinds of potential differences within and between the groups. That is, there is still a great deal of variety within the three family types, including, for example, the duration of conflict, the partners to conflict, time since divorce, and so forth.

The Comparative Divorce Groups Design

A third design attends to significant features of the postdivorce situation, thus addressing the problem of assuming uniform effects after divorce. In these designs children in different custody situations are compared, always with each other and sometimes with children from families with no divorce. These designs derive from the observation that divorce is a process that may take different forms, with different consequences for individuals and for families. Research employing these designs has produced significant information about the different implications for boys and girls of father- and mother-custody situations, complicating any notion of a uniform response to parental divorce and reminding us of the gendered nature of both divorcing and intact families. At the same time, studies using these designs (like the preceding ones) highlight one feature of the postdivorce family (custody) and ignore other kinds of differences.

The Within-Group Longitudinal Design

A final design frequently employed by researchers interested in parental divorce is longitudinal study of those affected by parental divorce (a within-group design). Studies employing this kind of design assume that the impact of parental divorce may not be uniform over time, and thus they have produced valuable information about the reduction in adjustment difficulties with distance in time from the divorce. In principle, studies of this sort can include comparison with those never affected by parental divorce. In practice, this is rarely done, partly because longitudinal designs highlight the fact that parental divorce produces, over time, other potential experiences not available to those in families where there has been no divorce (living in a single-parent household, having a stepparent, having stepsiblings, etc.), which also differentiate some of those affected by parental divorce from others so affected. Thus, longitudinal studies of parental divorce tend to focus on differences among individuals or families affected by parental divorce. However, these studies generally do assume that divorce is the critical event of psychological importance in the lives of the individuals studied. As a result, adjustment difficulties are sometimes attributed to the divorce, despite the lack of a relevant design for drawing this conclusion.

This last type of study, like most of the preceding ones, has often focused on the impact of parental divorce on individuals. Relatively little research using any of these designs assesses aspects of the divorce experience at other levels—such as the household or the dyadic level—or connects events at those levels with individual adjustment (see Ahrons, 1987; Camara & Resnick, 1987; Hetherington, 1989; Hetherington, et al., 1977; and Kurdek, 1987, for important exceptions).

A DESIGN FOR OUR STUDY

Because we were interested in the different experiences of families following parental divorce, we adopted a within-group design. We were not interested in assessing the impact of parental divorce itself on adjustment. We were, however, interested in understanding something about what parental divorce means to both adults and children. Because we assumed that divorce was a process, we knew that, over time, parental divorce might well recede in individuals' consciousness and also in its day-to-day importance, overshadowed by other important events. Therefore, we sampled families in which divorce was likely to be a prominent feature of daily life and of consciousness, and followed these families over the course of the divorcing process. Our time perspective is short (18 months from parental separation), in part because we knew that children's growth and development might confuse the picture by producing changes having nothing to do with adjustment to parental separation. We also knew that the rate of significant postdivorce changes (remarriage, moves, etc.) is very rapid, and adjustment to those changes could also confuse the picture.

We assessed families at different levels—the individual, the dyad, the whole family—because we were concerned with the relations among the different levels of change going on in divorcing families. One critical difference between families experiencing parental divorce and families in which no divorce has occurred may be that divorcing families are undergoing a *transformation* of the family structure within which they operate. Families in which there has been no divorce do experience other transformations due to, for example, additions of new siblings, additions and departures of extended family members from the household, and departures of adult children. Most of these changes, though, do not involve change in the parental dyad. Only death of a parent, or inclusion of a new "coparent" in the parental dyad, would. Future research may be able to address the differences and similarities among various kinds of family transformations.

Given our focus on the differences among divorcing families in the process of family transformation, we included attention to features of the custodial and noncustodial households, particular dyads (parent–parent and parent–child), and individuals. In addition, by thinking of the families as undergoing transformation rather than being in crisis, we could consider the possibility not only of adjustment difficulties, but of growth and development.

Even with our focus on within-group differences, a comparative design could have allowed us to explore the degree to which relationships we might find (e.g., between family experiences and adjustment) held in both families with and without divorces, or only in one. This is, we think, a potentially interesting question. However, making that comparison would require the assumption (discussed above) that parental divorce was the only or crucial difference between the two groups, and we were not at all sure we could safely make that assumption. More narrowly, we were not at all sure how to select a nondivorce sample that would constitute a useful comparison. Should we "match" families on social status and predivorce violence or might changes in status and violence be a part of the process of parental divorce—at least for some families? If that is the case, how then do we sample comparison families? We could choose families from among children's classmates, but what if (following divorce) the children's schools have changed? Should we select from among new classmates or old ones? From our perspective, and given our interests, the risk of misattributing any discovered differences to parental divorce, when they were really associated with some other difference between divorcing and currently intact families (such as amount of recent change in residence, work, school, and social network), was much greater than the potential knowledge to be gained by making comparisons.

Obviously, then, our conceptual framework had implications for our design. Our design and our assessment strategy—as in all other studies—has obscured some things from our view. We offer the knowledge generated by our approach with confidence that the knowledge generated by other approaches will enrich and complement it![1]

RECRUITING THE FAMILIES FOR OUR STUDY

In order to seek a sample of "divorcing families," it was important that we define what "divorcing" would mean for our purposes. Is it best defined in terms of the moment when an individual forms the intention of divorce? Or when a couple agrees to divorce? Or when one person physically leaves? Or when they take a legal action? Or when the divorce is "final"? There are usually at least a couple of years, and sometimes quite a few, from the first of these events to the last, so the definition surely matters! In addition, we know that many divorces are preceded by informal, physical separations that do not result in immediate divorce. Keeping in mind that our study aimed to explore the psychological meaning of divorce to both children and their parents, we defined divorce in terms that seemed likely to involve a high rate of permanent family changes and to be very meaningful to all family members.

Both an individual's intention and legal finality might be very meaningful to an adult, but completely invisible to a child. In contrast, the physical departure of one member of the couple would, we thought, be highly observable and meaningful to all members of a family experiencing parental divorce. Our desire to identify families in which the parents were separated and in the process of divorce (i.e., unlikely to reconcile) led to our sampling procedure.

The families in our study were recruited through a search of public divorce dockets of five counties in the greater Boston area. When individuals wished to pursue a divorce in Massachusetts during the 1980s, they initiated the legal process by stating their intention to dissolve their marriage in the court of the county in which they resided. When they filed that statement, they were asked to indicate whether they were living separately from their spouse, and if so for how long, as well as whether there were minor children involved, and their names and ages. Because the dockets were public records, we were able to use them to identify families in which physical separation had occurred within the past 6 months, and in which there was at least one child between the ages of 6 and 12 (who was designated the "focus child" for the study).

We chose families with at least one child of this age for several reasons. First, we wanted families in which child rearing would continue to be an issue for a substantial period of time; for these families custody and visitation arrangements would require children and their parents to negotiate a transition from a one-household to a two-household, partially overlapping family structure (see Ahrons, 1980, 1995). Second, we wanted to be able to interview the children, in order to get their perspective directly, so we felt it was important to sample families with at least one child old enough to articulate a point of view verbally.

Finally, because families were expected to drive to Boston University we only sampled families living no more than about 1 hour's drive from Boston. Because we were interested in differences among divorcing families, we placed no other constraints on the sample.

Both parties to the divorce were contacted by letter and asked to participate in our study. Those who indicated an interest were contacted by telephone, and an appointment was made for us to interview as many of the household members as possible. During this first, early postseparation period, at least one member of a total of 160 families (including 121 mothers and 57 fathers) agreed to participate in our study, which was about one-quarter of those we contacted. Of these, 24 families were represented only by a noncustodial father; in these cases, the custodial parent was not interested in participating. There were 103 families represented by custodial mothers and their children, but not the noncustodial father; 15 families were represented by custodial fathers and their children (and in 6 cases the noncustodial mothers participated too). Finally, in 18 families, both the custodial mother and the noncustodial father participated, as did the children. A total of 24 families participated in which both parents were interviewed. At least one child was interviewed from 136 families. See Table 2.2 for a summary of the sample.

Analyses presented in later chapters focus on different groups of mothers, fathers, children, dyads, and families. Therefore no absolute figures can be provided describing the numbers of individuals or families described in all analyses. Broadly speaking, though, the "core longitudinal sample" is comprised of those who participated both in the initial assessment and in the follow-up 1 year later. The two couples who participated at both times and reconciled during this period were, of course, not included. The resulting sample of families who participated both times, and were either divorced or still pursuing a divorce by the time of the follow-up, includes 103 families in which custodial or noncustodial mothers and their children participated, and 46 fathers (some of whom were not connected with the mothers and children in the sample). In particular chapters other groupings of participants are defined to address particular issues. In addition to variations according to the group being studied, sample sizes also fluctuate slightly because of missing data for any particular measure.

Descriptive information about the individuals and the families is contained in the next chapter. For the moment it may be sufficient to note that the sample is quite varied with respect to income, education, religion, and grounds for divorce. Moreover, unlike studies that depend on participants' involvement with clinical settings, our sample includes people who have never sought nor received professional counseling.

An important question to consider is how representative our sample is of divorcing families in the Boston area. We carried out some analyses of court docket data from several months in an effort to address this issue. We compared four groups: those who agreed to participate in our study; those

TABLE 2.2. Participants in the Family Changes Project

Families

103 custodial mothers and children
18 custodial mothers, noncustodial fathers, and children
6 noncustodial mothers, custodial fathers, and children
9 custodial fathers and children
24 noncustodial fathers only
160 families (142 at Time 2)

Mothers

103 custodial mothers, without participating fathers
18 custodial mothers, with participating fathers
6 noncustodial mothers, with participating fathers
127 mothers (110 at Time 2)

Fathers

24 noncustodial fathers, without participating mothers
18 noncustodial fathers, with participating mothers
9 custodial fathers, without participating mothers
6 custodial fathers, with participating mothers
57 fathers (42 at Time 2)

Focus children

103 with custodial mothers
18 with custodial mothers and noncustodial fathers
9 with custodial fathers
6 with custodial fathers and noncustodial mothers
136 focus children (102 at Time 2)

Note. At Time 2, seven couples had reconciled or remarried each other. We did not include them in the follow-up sample, although they were included in the Time 1 sample.

who met the criteria for participation but were never successfully reached (probably because their address had changed after the filing); those who met the criteria but refused to participate; and those who met our family stage criterion (having at least one child between 6 and 12 years old), but had been separated longer than 6 months (here we were interested in whether the time restriction biased the sample in any detectable way). Data were available to explore representativeness in terms of type of community of residence (urban, semiurban, suburban, and rural) and seven marital and family characteristics (number of children, age and sex of oldest and youngest child, number of months married, number of months separated). Eleven divorce-related variables were also coded (grounds for the divorce; motions for several kinds of court orders at the time of filing, including restraining, financial, child-related or other motions; whether custody was contested; whether there was a cross-complaint; whether there were postfiling motions of each kind).[2]

There were no differences on any of these variables between those who participated and either of the other groups meeting the criteria for participation (those we never reached and those who refused). There were some differences between participants and those who had been separated too long for inclusion in the study. Of course they differed in number of months separated; those who had been separated longer than our sample were involved in fewer postfiling legal motions (though not fewer legal actions of any other kind). Perhaps, then, by selecting families that filed for separation and/or divorce rather quickly after physical separation, we increased the likelihood that we included families in which legal conflict was more intense or more protracted.

One variable that was not available to us in the court records was the race or ethnicity of family members. This fact is of concern to us because our procedure produced only a small number of families in which at least one parent was not of European American descent (about 5%). Given the demographic composition of the communities we were sampling from, we had hoped for a sample that reflected greater ethnic diversity. On the basis of community characteristics, we had especially anticipated more participation by African American families. Because the public records did not include information about race we were unable adequately to explore the reasons for the low representation of African American families. However, we suspect that it was the unintended consequence of our dependence on legal records and one of our sampling criteria, namely recent physical separation.

It has been noted repeatedly that African Americans are less likely to marry than European Americans and are more likely to divorce (Norton & Glick, 1979; Price & McKenry, 1988; Walker, 1988). If African Americans do divorce, though, they are likely to do so after long physical separations (Norton & Glick, 1979). By limiting our sample to those recently separated, we probably oversampled those with a tendency to seek legal sanction for their actions, and thereby undersampled African Americans. No doubt we also undersampled other groups with reservations about the legal system (e.g., immigrants). Moreover, although our sample is diverse with respect to family income and definitely includes families experiencing economic hardship, we suspect that it must nevertheless be somewhat skewed toward the upper end, because at least one parent had to have either the economic resources or the confidence to file legal papers. A future study of family transformation could and should be defined in terms of exploration of the impact of physical separation (rather than legal filing for divorce); such a study could employ a potentially more inclusive sampling approach (e.g., "snowball" sampling within communities, a method permitting participants to suggest other potential participants they know).

It is also true that by defining family transformation in terms of legal marriage, we did not include any gay or lesbian families in this study. Just as there are an increasing number of studies of gay and lesbian parents and families, there is a need for research on the impact of dissolution of intimate partnerships in those families. Again, a different recruitment strategy is required for such a study.

CHARACTERISTICS OF THE FAMILIES IN OUR STUDY

Obviously all of our participating families lived in the Greater Boston area; most family members were born in New England. As mentioned before, they were mostly European American. Half of our participants were Catholic; most of the rest, Protestant. They varied widely in social class: the average sample family was lower-middle to middle class, about a fourth were working poor or unemployed, and a few were professionals. The couples had been married for an average of 12 years, and for most (over 85%) this was their first marriage. About half had experienced at least one previous separation in this marriage.

Because of the criteria for participation in the study, all families had at least one elementary school-age child; over a third also had a preschool-age child, and over a fourth had an adolescent child. Thirteen percent of the children were from a previous marriage. Two-thirds of the families had no more than three children, and there were equal proportions of boys and girls. Following the separation, most children lived with their mother, generally with no other adult. An additional adult resided in 13% of the postseparation households, usually a relative, a boarder, or a lover. At the time of initial contact, almost all of our participating mothers had sole or physical custody of their children; 1 year later, four children's living arrangements had changed. (In Massachusetts "legal" custody was defined by decision-making authority over the child; "physical" custody by the child's residence. "Sole" custody includes both. In many cases, parents shared legal custody, but mothers had physical custody.) Almost half of the participating fathers had sole or physical custody. A little over 10% of the total sample were father-custody families, about the same as the national rate (see Emery 1988).

Overall, the sample is reasonably representative of divorcing families with school-age children in the greater Boston area in the 1980s. The rate of Catholic families is certainly higher than in many parts of the United States, but is characteristic of the Boston area. It is important to recall that there is substantial variety within the groups identified as either "Catholic" or "non-Catholic."

The fact that the study was conducted in the 1980s must certainly have played a role in influencing participants' responses to divorce. Although we have no direct comparative data from other periods, we note that divorce rates in the United States generally rose until 1988, when they plateaued, perhaps even beginning to fall (National Center for Health Statistics, 1989; Rice, 1994). Although divorce laws were generally made less restrictive during the 1960s and 1970s, probably reflecting increased social acceptability of divorce (Thornton, 1989), at least by the early 1990s public discourse about divorce was quite critical and more restrictive legislation was proposed and passed (see, e.g., Popenoe, 1993, for a scholarly critique; Whitehead, 1993, for an influential popular one; see also Rice, 1994, and Stacey, 1991, for analyses of this antidivorce feeling). Our study, then, took place during the period in which divorce was relatively frequent; in addition, it took place at what may have been the peak in divorce's acceptability to the American public. Our findings must, then, be understood as arising within a particular historical context.

On the other hand, there is evidence that historical period has limited and quite specific effects on findings in divorce research. Amato and Keith (1991) assessed the degree to which the year in which a study was conducted (1950–1969; 1970–1979; 1980–1989) affected the study's findings, in terms of seven "outcomes" of divorce for children: academic achievement, conduct, psychological adjustment, self-concept, social adjustment, mother–child relations, and father–child relations. For four of these the year of the study played no role at all; for three of them (academic achievement, conduct, and mother–child relations) it did play a role, in all cases in the direction of weaker effects of divorce in the later periods. This suggests that as acceptability and frequency increased, divorce had fewer negative effects on children's adjustment. Our goal, though, is not to estimate the overall impact of divorce, but to explore variations in the kinds of impact. These variations probably persist even when the overall impact lessens. Moreover, our focus in this book is substantially on areas that did not show the influence of history (psychological adjustment, self-concept, social adjustment, and father–child relations).

The fact that our study involved participants sampled in Massachusetts may also be an important issue. We have already noted that in the Boston area a higher proportion of families are Catholic than in other areas. Our sample is also relatively urban and suburban. It may be important that this study was conducted in the Northeast, in contrast with other studies conducted in California (Wallerstein & Blakeslee, 1989), the South (Hetherington, 1987), or the Midwest (Ahrons, 1995; Kitson, 1992). It is hard to know exactly how region would affect the results, except perhaps in the relative rate of divorce within the immediate area of study participants. This is rarely, or never, reported and would be difficult to define. Thus, is the critical issue the rate of divorce in the participant's own neighborhood or town, the region as a whole, a child's school district? Is it important to break the rate down by age, income, racial/ethnic group, or education? Perhaps the most important issue is the legal context of divorce, which certainly varies state by state (and over time). In Massachusetts, at the time of the study, no-fault divorce was available as an option to divorcing couples. We suspect that the legal context is one important way in which the location of studies matters, so we examine the different kinds of divorces (fault and no-fault) our families pursued and obtained.

Finally, it should be noted that a far larger proportion of mothers participated than fathers. For that reason, we have more confidence in the representativeness of our samples of mothers and children than of fathers. In addition, noncustodial fathers were particularly unlikely to participate in the study; a far higher percentage of participating fathers were custodial parents (almost half) than the rate of custodial father households in the entire sample (10%). Despite the relatively lower confidence we have in the representativeness of the father sample, we have retained it in the analyses, because we felt it was so important to include men's perspective on this family experience.

The parents in our study ranged in age from 22 to 56, with an average age of 34 for the mothers and 38 for the fathers. Most of the women had married at about age 22, though a few married in their teens and a few when they were in their 30s. The average age at marriage for the men was 27. Most of our participants grew up in two-parent families of origin (though nearly 25% had experienced their own parents' divorce). Most of the mothers had finished high school, but only about one-fifth had graduated from college; very few held graduate degrees. Over 90% of the fathers had completed high school, over one-fifth had college degrees but no further education, and two-fifths had some graduate training.

Half of the mothers were employed outside the home both before and after the separation, two-fifths full-time. Seventeen percent increased their work hours after the separation, and another 25% entered the labor market for the first time since having children. Overall, then, more than three-fourths of the mothers were employed in the initial period following the separation, two-thirds of whom worked more than 20 hours per week. Only about 10% did not work at all outside the home either before or after the separation, usually because they were caring for very young children. All but one of the fathers were employed at the initial data collection, although 50% had experienced a significant job change in the 2 years prior to the first interview.

OUR PROCEDURES

Parents who agreed to participate in the study were sent a packet of questionnaires about themselves and one of their children. If they only had one child between the ages of 6 and 12, that child was designated the "focus" child for our study; if there was more than one 6- to 12-year-old we arbitrarily designated one as the "focus" child, maintaining roughly equal numbers of boys and girls of each age. Questionnaires were included assessing aspects of the family structure and history; parents' own emotional, physical, and social adjustment; their parenting style; and their perceptions of the adjustment of the focus child. We asked parents to complete the questionnaires and bring them to an interview session, along with their children. We interviewed any children above age 5 who were living at home and were willing to be interviewed, and provided child care for younger children.

Before the interviews, the family group was given an explanation of what would happen and was shown the various interview rooms (so children and their parents would understand each other's whereabouts). Each family member was then asked to sign an informed consent form, which included explicit mention of the fact that what was said in the interview would not be repeated to any other family member. Family members were interviewed separately, with children usually interviewed in playrooms and parents usually interviewed in project offices. Parent interviews lasted about 1½ to 2 hours. Parents were asked about various aspects of family life since the separation and about the history of their marriage and the separation. They were also asked to talk about the focus child's personality, reactions to the separation, relationships with all family members, experience with visiting the noncustodial parent, other important experiences before and since the separation, and school, home, and physical adjustment. In addition, some questions were asked about the other children.

After the interviews, parents were given a "resource packet" we developed. It included information about general resources for families experiencing stresses (counseling, financial, etc.) and for families experiencing divorce per se (groups for children and divorce, associations of single parents, etc.). Parents were also asked if we could contact their children's teachers. Virtually all of them said yes, and teachers were sent the Teacher Form of the Achenbach Child Behavior Checklist (CBCL; Edelbrock & Achenbach, 1984); 83% returned them. Parents were asked at the same time if they were willing to return for a videotaped play/interaction session. If they agreed, an effort was made to schedule the return visit within a couple of weeks.

Children were interviewed for approximately 30 to 45 minutes. They were asked about their daily routines, family members, and their perceptions of and feelings about their parents' separation. After the interviews, the children were given a 15-minute break, during which they were given a small snack and were able to play with the toys available in the room. After the break, several standard questionnaires were read to them, and their responses were recorded. These questionnaires usually took about 30 minutes to administer. The procedure for adolescent children (13 and older) was similar to that for younger children, but they were asked to complete the questionnaires in writing rather than orally.

About half of the mother-custody families returned for the second play/interaction session. (Table 2.3 lists our different contacts with the families.) Because there were so few father-custody families in the sample, and the rate of agreement to participate in this session was about 50%, we felt any sample of father-custody families would be too small for analysis. Therefore we only collected play/interaction data from mother-custody families. (The 53 who agreed to participate the first year did not differ from the 50 nonparticipating families on any of the psychological variables assessed in the mothers or children, nor did they differ on demographic variables such as age, length of marriage, number of months separated, etc. Thus we feel confident that the participating families are representative of the larger sample of mother-custody families.) Families were again given an explanation of the session, showed the video camera, and asked to sign an informed consent form. Mothers played (in a structured session) alone with the focus child for 30 minutes. When the focus child had a sibling between 5 and 14 years old,

TABLE 2.3. Overview of Family Changes Project

First year

- Mailed letters to parents identified from court documents, asking for their participation.
- Mailed packet of questionnaires to all parents agreeing to participate in the study.
- Mothers and fathers (both with and without children) participated in interviews at Boston University.
- Mailed feedback questionnaire to all parent participants.
- Mailed questionnaire to children's teachers (with parental consent).
- Mothers and their children returned to Boston University for videotaped play/interaction sessions.

Second year

- Mailed packet of questionnaires to all parents agreeing to participate in the follow-up study.
- Mothers and fathers (both with and without children) participated in interviews at Boston University.
- Mailed feedback questionnaire to all parent participants; designed to permit anonymous return.
- Mailed questionnaire to children's teachers (with parental consent).
- Mothers and their children returned to Boston University for videotaped play/interaction sessions.

the two children also played together for 30 minutes. In each case, a video camera (which had been pointed out, but was partially camouflaged), was left recording in the room; no project staff members were present.

Prior to the mother–child play session, mothers were given instructions for the whole 30-minute period, without the child hearing. Briefly, they were told that for 10 minutes they should play with a few preselected toys; no specific instructions about how or what to play were given. At the end of that time, a project staff member would briefly enter the room and suggest that they go on to the second activity, which was tower building. In a task adapted from Rosen and D'Andrade (1959), children tried to build a high tower of wooden blocks while blindfolded. Mothers were told they could help in any way they wished. It was suggested that this task continue for about 10 more minutes, but mothers could decide when to stop. For the remainder of the time, mothers and children made a puppet or mask together from paper bags, socks, paper plates, and other craft supplies.

Families were paid a modest sum for their participation in each session and were told we would contact them within a year for a follow-up. After the interview session, parents were sent a thank-you letter, and an anonymous feedback questionnaire asking for the family's reactions to the interview.

During the second year, the procedures we followed were identical, though the interviews were slightly shorter, because they did not include a second account of the preseparation period. Ninety-two percent of the mothers and 84% of the fathers returned for the follow-up. It should be noted, though, that all of the custodial fathers returned. Thus, the return rate for noncustodial fathers (as for the much smaller sample of noncustodial mothers) was only 80%.

FAMILIES' VIEWS OF THEIR PARTICIPATION

We knew that many of the participating families were already quite stressed, and we couldn't know in advance what effects participating in the study might have. Therefore, we sought feedback a couple of weeks after the interviews, and tried to provide parents with freedom to be critical. We asked parents to comments on their own and their children's feelings, by returning a questionnaire containing no identifying information. While we hoped that participation might be beneficial—perhaps in providing a neutral context in which to talk about a painful experience—it seemed important to create an opportunity to find out about it if participation was, in fact, upsetting or harmful. After the first round of interviews, 71 people returned our questionnaire and after the second, 67 did. All adults were asked, "How would you describe your own reaction to participating in the research project?" and parents who brought children in were also asked, "How would you describe your child(ren)'s reaction(s) to participating in the research project?" In both years, responses to these questions were overwhelmingly positive. While some parents felt the questionnaires we had asked them to complete before coming in were too time consuming, they also generally found them interesting, or could see why they might be valuable. Parents also enjoyed their interview sessions, with the vast majority commenting that they were "interesting" and "enjoyable," and that they were happy to participate in the hope that the study would eventually be helpful to others.

A substantial minority expressed stronger feelings about the value, to them, of participating in the interviews. One theme that emerged was that the opportunity to talk was therapeutic; for example, one woman said, "It was a relief to have someone objective ask questions and be able to respond about personal feelings in a nonjudgmental environment." Another theme was the opportunity the interview and questionnaires provided for self-reflection; for example, "I thoroughly enjoyed participating in the research project—it showed me how far I had come and I got to know myself much better." Another mother wrote, "I was nervous at first but after awhile I found it comfortable. To talk about what had happened between my husband and myself and my children gave me some perspective on what went wrong."

Many parents also mentioned that participation provided an outing for them and their children, and that the occasion opened up new opportunities to talk together about the divorce. One mother wrote, "It brought up many different conversations between the children and myself," while another indicated that

> "it was a very good opportunity for my children and I to do something together as a family. Also, my son and I were able to discuss questions and feelings after our interview session, which was great! We haven't really talked too much about the separation. . . . My initial reaction to the study was not to take part in it, but I'm glad that I changed my mind."

Parents indicated that they thought children responded very positively, though perhaps with less understanding. (Probably this was more true of younger children, but because the questionnaires were deliberately anonymous we have no way to be sure.) For example, one mother said, "They didn't quite understand it but enjoyed 'play' in a different place." Particular themes that arose in the parents' descriptions of children's reactions included the parents' sense that "having someone interested in their feelings made them feel important." In addition, some parents felt that children had previously been afraid to, but "needed to talk about what happened." Several mentioned that for their children participation in the project demonstrated that "he isn't the only child with divorced parents" and that was helpful.

After participation the second year, many parents reported a sense of "completion." In response to the question about their reactions to the interview, one parent wrote that she enjoyed being able

> "to relate all the changes in a year and realize that my motivation was different this year. Last year I was interested in the money to do something with my kids for the day. This year, to have a sense of completeness that the old life was truly gone."

Another mentioned, "It gave me an opportunity to examine what I've accomplished in the past year—and realize how far I've come!" In the second year children were described as less apprehensive about coming in ("Very positive, no fear or anxiety this time"), and otherwise the same themes emerged:

> "My children enjoyed feeling important, knowing that someone cared enough to talk to them about this, that someone thought their reactions and opinions actually mattered. Not having their feelings pushed aside has been a great help."

Overall, though, the single most frequent theme, mentioned often both years, was the desire to help others who would experience parental divorce. While a handful of people did not find that project participation was particularly satisfying, none reported any negative effects. Overall, responses reassured us that the project was not doing harm. While it is clearly possible that participation in the project actually supported families' adjustment after divorce, we feel it would be grandiose and inaccurate to view this project as a major intervention in this long and complex process.

DESCRIPTION OF KEY MEASURES

Obviously we obtained an enormous amount of data from questionnaires, interviews, observations of structured play, and legal records. We obtained those data from as many family members as we could in each family. In this book we can only hope to report on some of the interesting aspects of the data. One strategy we have used to help avoid overloading the reader with methodological information in any one part of the book is to introduce new information about measures in each chapter, as they are being used or discussed for the first time. In this chapter, then, we will not describe every measure used but will limit ourselves to those measures of individual adjustment and adaptation ("well-being") that are used throughout the book. Then each chapter can introduce those measures that have not been covered before.

Children's Adjustment and Well-Being

Because we viewed children's adjustment and well-being as multifaceted, including their emotional responses, physical symptoms, and behavior in a variety of settings and in the eyes of themselves, their parents, and their teachers, we included a number of assessments of it. We knew that children might reveal different types of responses in different situations. For example, a child who was quite distressed about the family situation might throw herself into schoolwork or peer activities, showing few negative signs in these arenas. However, that same child might develop headaches and stomachaches.

Similarly, different people might have different interpretations of a child's behavior; for example, a mother who never sees her child cry might report that the child is not especially sad. The child, knowing he cries alone at night might, in contrast, report that he is very sad. Or a mother might report that a child was acting up in school, while a child might indicate that she is doing fine in school. Although the mother's report in this case may be more "objective" or factually correct about the child's behavior, the child's self-acceptance might be the more important indicator of the child's adjustment.

We assessed three different areas of children's adjustment and well-being with four well-validated measures: psychological adjustment (children's report), behavior problems (mother and teacher report), and physical illness (mother report). In the area of psychological adjustment, three scores obtained from children themselves were combined to create an overall index. First, children completed two standard psychological measures: the Perceived Competence Scale (Harter, 1982), which provided an overall indication of self-perceived social competence, or self-esteem; and an adaptation for children of the Twenty Symptoms measure (Veroff, Kulka, & Douvan, 1981), which assesses psychological and physical symptoms often associated with stress (e.g., bad dreams, difficulty sleeping, headaches, loss of appetite).

In addition to these standard measures, an assessment of children's feelings, or affect, about their parent's separation was developed for this study and included in the composite index. Children were asked, "How do you feel about your parents' separation (or divorce, if appropriate)?" Open-ended responses to this question were then coded as present or absent for feelings of surprise, confusion, sadness, responsibility or guilt, global distress, fear, anger, relief, and gladness. After the child's response to the open-ended question, the interviewer said:

> "It's usually very hard for people to describe exactly how they feel—partly because sometimes they feel a lot of different things at the same time. I'm going to read you a list of things that kids sometimes feel when their parents are getting separated, and for each of these I'd like you to

tell me if you feel that way about your parents getting separated a lot, a little, or not at all. Some kids feel sad. Do you feel that way a lot, a little, or not at all?"

The last question was then repeated for the following divorce-related feelings: angry, confused, glad, scared, surprised, like it's partly their fault. A total negative emotion score was created by treating open-ended report of an emotion as adding 1 point to the 3-point scales (1 = not at all, 2 = a little, 3 = a lot, 4 = open-ended mention plus closed-ended rating of "a lot") and then summing positive emotions (glad, relieved) and subtracting them from the sum of negative ones (sad, scared, confused, angry, surprised, like it's partly their fault).[3]

Both custodial parents and teachers were asked to provide ratings of children's behavior problems on the Parent and Teacher Forms of the widely cited Child Behavior Checklist (CBCL; Achenbach, 1978; Achenbach & Edelbrock, 1978; Edelbrock & Achenbach, 1984). Although both scales can yield a large number of subscales, the subscales were highly intercorrelated in this sample, so we restricted ourselves to the overall scores for behavior problems. Parent and teacher ratings of behavior problems were significantly correlated both years. Finally, custodial parents reported on their children's physical health on a questionnaire that drew together items from several available sources (Wahler, 1973; Abramson, Terepolsky, Brook, & Kark, 1965). The total number of common illnesses (e.g., headaches, stomachaches, colds) reported during the previous 3 months provided our mother-report measure of children's physical health.[4]

Parents' Adjustment and Well-Being

As with children, we employed several relatively standard questionnaires with parents, designed to tap different domains of adjustment. These included indicators of psychological adjustment (including mood disturbance, life satisfaction, self-esteem, and stress symptoms) and physical health.

In order to assess parents' overall mood (paralleling children's divorce-related feelings), we first used the Profile of Mood States (POMS; McNair, Lorr, & Droppleman, 1971), a 65-item checklist of emotions. Each parent rated the frequency of experiencing each feeling over the past few months. The POMS yields separate scores for six subscales (anger, tension, depression, fatigue, confusion, and vigor). In addition, an overall index of "mood disturbance" is created by summing scores on the first five scales, and subtracting the vigor scale score. Many studies have demonstrated that the POMS significantly differentiates a variety of emotionally distraught clinical samples from samples of adults not experiencing distress, and that it is sensitive to changes in levels of emotional disturbance (see McNair, Lorr, & Droppleman, 1971, for a review of validity studies).

As a measure of self-acceptance paralleling the children's self-report, we included the self-esteem scale developed by Rosenberg (1965). The scale is a 10-item test that has been widely used and well validated. Each parent completed the questionnaire on stress symptoms based on Gurin, Veroff, and Feld's (1960) and Veroff and colleagues' (1981) national study of mental health in American adults. Finally, in order to assess global well-being, we included in our questionnaires a single 4-point item on which parents rated how satisfied they were with their lives. Possible responses ranged from "completely satisfied" to "not very satisfied." Robinson, Shaver, and Wrightsman (1991) provide validational evidence from two national surveys that substantiate the use of this kind of item as a measure of general life satisfaction. The four indicators were significantly correlated with each other at both times, so we combined them to create one overall index of psychological adjustment.[5]

For our second adult adjustment measure, parents, like children, were asked to indicate whether they had experienced a variety of common ailments over the preceding 3 months. These included headaches, stomachaches, colds, and flu. An overall index of physical illnesss was created by totaling reported illnesses. Over time, these reports were quite stable.[6] The only aspect of psychological adjustment that was significantly correlated with physical illness reports was stress symptoms, and only in the first year.

THE REST OF THIS BOOK

Two overarching concerns shape the chapters to come. First, what is the course of the period following parental separation like for families, for children, and for their custodial and noncustodial parents? This question will be addressed first (in Chapters 3 and 4) by describing the explicit comments our participants made about the process. It will, however, also be addressed by examining changes in various kinds of scores over time in all of the remaining chapters. The statistics used for assessing change include matched *t*-tests and repeated measures analyses of variance. Both of these analyses will help us identify differences in scores that suggest reliable or dependable changes over time.

The second major concern is with understanding the factors that make a difference in adjustment and well-being, either for a group as a whole, or for subgroups within it. Thus, the next six chapters will focus on particular groups (parents in Chapter 5, children in Chapter 6, mother–child dyads in Chapter 7, parental dyads in Chapters 8 and 9, and families in Chapter 10). Within each of these chapters, factors that seemed to help or hinder adaptation overall will be identified; in addition, factors that helped or hindered the adaptation of some, but not all, subgroups will also be discussed (e.g., boys but not girls; mothers employed outside the home, but not those at home full-time; poorer families, but not more affluent ones; etc.). Moreover, within each chapter we will separately consider the factors that were important in the early postseparation period, the ones that seemed to matter over time (between the early and the later period), and the ones that only seemed to matter during the later period. The usual statistical procedures employed in these chapters include correlations and multiple regressions, with the adjustment and well-being scores described in this chapter treated as "dependent" or outcome variables. These analyses will help us identify the factors that make an important, independent contribution to the adjustment or well-being of individuals, dyads, and families. In addition, we will draw liberally from interviews, sometimes including extensive case materials or formal content analysis, often quoting from particularly illuminating transcripts.

Finally, in Chapter 11, we will draw some conclusions about the process involved in family transformation as a result of parental separation—for individuals, for dyads, and for the family as a whole. Here we will attempt to assess not only what the results of this study have shown, but how they might be used to realize our participating families' hope (and our own) that, as one of the mothers said, this study "will be helpful to those people who are going through or may go through separation and divorce."

NOTES

1. We note that the other large study most similar to ours is Ahrons (1995). Both involve examination of the divorce process over time in nonclinical samples of families with minor children. Differences include timing (Ahrons studied her couples at 1, 3, and 5 years after the divorce; we began within 6 months of the physical separation and ended 1 year later), location (her sample was from Wisconsin, ours from Boston), inclusion of children as participants (we did, she didn't), age of children in family (she included families if there were any minor children; we included only families with at least one child between 6 and 12), and involvement of fathers in the postdivorce family (she restricted her sample to families in which fathers were very involved; we did not).

2. We used analyses of variance and chi-squares, as appropriate, to test for differences among the groups on these variables.

3. Intercorrelations were high, $p < .001$; the three scores were standard-scored before combining.

4. All of the adjustment and well-being indicators showed over-time stability (correlations ranging from $r = .30$, $p < .001$, for physical health reports, to $r = .76$, $p < .001$, for mother-rated behavior problems). In addition, although mother and teacher ratings of children's behavior problems were significantly correlated both years, $r = .33$, $p < .01$,

and $r = .46$, $p < .001$, the other indicators were mostly uncorrelated. Thus, the various indicators provide reliable and independent information about children's adjustment and well-being.

5. All of the variables showed some stability over time; correlations ranged from $r = .34$, $p < .01$, for life satisfaction, to $r = .68$, $p < .001$, for psychological symptoms. The four indicators were standard-scored before combining.

6. The correlation over time was $r = .70$, $p < .001$.

CHAPTER 3

The Parents' Stories
THE END OF A MARRIAGE
AND A NEW BEGINNING

The parents we met were eager to tell us the story of their marriages and divorces. These stories are important not because we can fully rely on them as accounts of what "really" happened, but because they capture something of the texture of the experience of parental divorce for the people involved. They also offer a view of the complexity and diversity of the experience.

Certainly there was no one story that fit all the families in our study. At the same time, each story was not absolutely unlike every other story. In the first part of this chapter we will describe the parents' stories in terms of the most frequent themes that arose at each point in the "plot." Speaking most generally, a long period of marital difficulties ended with the husband or wife deciding that a separation would be best. A legal process followed, which varied in its duration and in the conflict involved. After the separation, most parents went through a period in which they faced many demands for active coping. They worked hard to meet these demands, often feeling inadequate to the situation and seeking help from others. Over time they developed more confidence and found that they were able to do what had to be done. By the end of the period of the study (18 months from the separation), they had developed a certain mastery over their situation and had high hopes for the future.

This is the narrative we heard from most, but not all, of the parents. There were some differences between men and women, and there were cer-

This chapter was drafted by Nia Lane Chester and Abigail J. Stewart.

tainly important exceptions. In this chapter, we will examine the stories in detail. At the end of the chapter, we will see how well their stories relate to a general theory of adaptation to changes.

Perhaps the most striking commonality among the parents' stories was that they began with an account of a long process of breakdown of the marriage. We had designed the study to begin near the beginning of one story (the transformation of the family from a one-household, two-parent structure to a two-household, single-parent structure); we were, however, also coming in at the end of the parents' story of their relationship. The fact that for parents these are two quite separate stories made their experience crucially different from that of their children. Although parents and children shared the experience of transforming their family life after the separation, before it parents had usually struggled with their marital difficulties in private.

STORIES OF MARRIAGES ENDING

The story of divorce, from the parents' point of view, inevitably began with the story of a marriage. In the case of these families that story reflected many years (an average of about 12) and a variety of life experiences, always including parenting. In some cases one person gradually recognized that the marriage could not be made to work; in others, both came to that recognition in a mutual process. In virtually every case, the loss of faith in the shared vision of marriage and family life was painful and protracted. Three-quarters of the mothers and fathers indicated that they had been thinking about separation and divorce for more than a year before the actual filing. In fact, half of the mothers indicated they had been thinking about it for more than 5 years. The divorces eventually pursued by these couples were, then, usually preceded by long periods of conflict or lonely alienation within the marriage. A few case studies—described without identifying details, using invented names— illustrate some of the different paths toward separation.

Persistent Violent Conflict: The Nelsons

When we met them, the Nelsons had been married 7 years and had three children, one a preschooler. Nora Nelson stayed home to care for the children; Ned Nelson worked in the financial department of a small company. The "screaming and yelling has been going on half our married life," said Nora. "The first time he hit me was when I was pregnant, and it just got worse." "Just your average amount of arguing," according to Ned. "Loud but cerebral, nothing physical." The Nelsons separated for the first time a year prior to filing for divorce. During that year they reconciled several times, but Nora also had to obtain a restraining order to keep her husband out of the home following a drunken and violent scene. On the final occasion, Ned moved in with friends with whom he had stayed during previous short separations and said he was going to speak to a lawyer. When he did not, Nora contacted one and filed for divorce.

Abuse of alcohol (and, to a lesser degree, other drugs) by at least one partner was mentioned as a problem in the marriage by close to half of the mothers and about a quarter of the fathers. Themes of physical violence arose in about one-quarter of the stories we heard (mothers were more likely to mention it than fathers). These violent stories reminded us that the decision to separate was often made at a point when the marital home had actually become a dangerous place. In some cases, the physical violence was described as having occurred only once, after the couple had been experiencing tension and conflict for some time; in others, the conflict escalated but the couple separated without any violent explosion.

Escalation of Conflict: The Elkins

Married for 10 years when we first interviewed her, Elaine Elkin had three children, all under age 7. Her husband, Eric, was a technician; Elaine stayed at home with the children, although she had worked until the birth of the second child. Over the years the Elkins' arguments increased, particularly about the cost and care of the children, as well as Elaine's feeling that her husband paid no attention to her. Elaine felt pressured by her husband to get a job, but she also felt she should stay home with the two youngest children. Their arguments about how to raise the children were based on beliefs and practices arising from their different cultural backgrounds. Elaine began having headaches and difficulty sleeping. During an argument about whether their daughter should be allowed to go to a birthday party at someone else's house, Eric hit Elaine. Shortly after this, she brought up the topic of separation ("He was always threatening to leave anyway," she said. "I was sure he was going to at some point."). Eric moved out 2 weeks later, and Elaine filed for divorce.

Many stories, with and without violent episodes, involved a process of gradual alienation of one or both of the partners. Over time, they recognized that the marriage simply was not meeting enough of their needs, despite the fact that as a couple they had weathered many difficulties. For example, over a third of the families described at least one child as having severe physical and/or emotional difficulties, including cerebral palsy, leukemia, and developmental delay. Sharing the worries and caretaking demands involved in raising these children bound the parents together, but also strained their resources for coping (see Seligman & Darling, 1997; Turk & Kerns, 1985).

Gradual Alienation: The Stones

Both the Stones worked full-time at professional-level jobs and were involved in the busy lives of their three children, one of whom had a chronic and serious disease (although he was mostly an energetic, active boy typical of his age). Although Sheldon felt their marriage had been relatively tranquil, Sheryl had felt for a long time (5 years, by her account) that there was little emotional content to their relationship and that her husband was not supportive of her efforts to redirect her career. She raised the subject of separation with Sheldon. "I was stunned and wouldn't agree at first," he said. "But finally there didn't seem much point to going on. But it's all from her, as far as I'm concerned."

In many cases, acceptance of the failure of the marriage was not so one sided; it often included strenuous individual and couple efforts to repair their strained relationship. Over 60% of the mothers and almost half of the fathers mentioned that at least one of them had been in counseling or psychotherapy at some time before the separation. About half of these experiences consisted of brief consultations with social workers and therapists, aimed at resolving marital or family difficulties. The other half were short- or longer-term psychotherapy. In some cases, counseling could not resolve the conflict parents felt in their visions of desirable marital roles; if one partner longed to move toward more egalitarian and similar roles, and the other remained committed to a more gender-differentiated model of marriage, only a separation could resolve the conflict.

Gender-Linked Marital Role Tension: The Crosslands

The Crosslands lived with their children in a household shared with other friends. Carol stayed home with the two children, devoting herself completely, both parents acknowledged, to her role as a mother, while Christopher worked as a high school teacher. As the children got older, Carol began to envy her husband's freedom and to feel constrained by the demands of constantly caring for the children. Christopher felt increasingly resentful of what he saw as her constant demands on him to take over with the children as soon as he walked in the door. "I work all day, and then I came home to more work. I always did as much as she did with the children and chores when I was home." He felt she alternated between wanting no interference with the children to wanting him to take care of them full-time so she could go back to school. When Carol did finally enter a degree program, the couple grew farther apart. "I looked at it as someday we could both be breadwinners and both be homemakers," commented Carol, "and that, you know, the roles wouldn't be so defined that one of us would be doing all of one and one of us all the other. But as the years went on and the kids got older it became more and more clear that he really didn't want the status to change." "I found it harder and harder to please her," said Christopher. "And I admit, I finally lost interest in trying." The Crosslands entered marriage counseling, but after a year they agreed that they should separate.

It is clear from these stories that separation and divorce did not result from a single decision, but a sequence of events and experiences taking place over a period of months or years. Of the images we encountered in Chapter 1 as characterizing previous thinking about divorce, the one most prominent in the accounts of the breakdown of the marriage was loss. Although feelings of sadness and despair were commonly described in this period, these feelings did not have either the intensity or the sudden onset that might characterize trauma. They were often accompanied by conflict as well; thus anger, resentment, and frustration were prominent emotions. Traditional psychological theory about loss, including traumatic loss, developed mostly to address losses that are unwelcome, sudden, and imposed from outside, such as bereavement and disasters. In the case of divorce for parents, the picture is more complicated. There is, of course, a great deal of loss: of a life partner, of companionship, of a way of life, a role, and a vision of the self in a family. However, these losses are accompanied by many other, sometimes contradictory, feelings: frustration at the failure of efforts to make things work, rage at the self and the partner for that failure, and hope that a better life may lie ahead of the current pain. In fact, the decision to separate and divorce can be seen as a strong indication of the belief that life could and may be better. For that reason, divorce cannot be fully characterized as loss, at least for adults.

Overall, then, the emotional process of divorce for parents was protracted and complex. Moreover, it was nearly impossible to define a beginning point. Most married people have moments of frustration, rage, and doubt about their marriage. For some, these moments become part of a coherent story of growing certainty that the marriage cannot be sustained, as well as actions that bring the marriage to an end. Even within a marriage the partners do not always reach a sense of certainty about the need to end their marriage at the same time. For parents, the first story, which Bohannon (1970) calls the "emotional divorce," is *not* like many other life changes (marriage, parenthood, entering the labor force) and losses (bereavement, disaster), which have a clear beginning followed by a process of adaptation.

UNDERSTANDING THE FAILURE OF THE MARRIAGE

In the first interview, we asked parents to describe for us both the kinds of problems and difficulties they had had in their marriage and what they thought was the "main reason" for the separation. From these accounts, we can see how parents understood what happened to their marriages.[1] It is important to remember that only a minority of the mothers and fathers we interviewed were married to each other. Most came from separate couples, and there were many more mothers than fathers in the study. Finally, a substantial proportion of the fathers and nearly all the mothers we interviewed had custody of their children.

Most mothers and fathers said that the major problems they faced in their marriage arose from specific behavior patterns of their spouse that they found intolerable (see Table 3.1 for exact percentages of parents reporting various problems). These negative behavior patterns included not being respectful or supportive, spending too many evenings out with friends, and generally not being committed to "family life" or to their responsibilities as a husband or wife. Other problems that were mentioned by more than a third of the parents included extramarital affairs; developing in different directions; money; child-related issues; lack of communication; irritating personality characteristics, such as inflexibility or immaturity; and serious behavior problems, such as alcoholism, emotional abuse, and psychological disorders. Finally, physical violence was mentioned as a problem in the marriage by almost a quarter of the mothers, but only a handful of the fathers. Obviously these problems were not mutually exclusive, and many parents mentioned several of these problems. This high level of reported difficulty in the marriage fits in well with our sense that the couples had struggled for a long time with minor and major problems and had only gradually concluded that the marriage could not be saved.

TABLE 3.1. Major Problems in the Marriage

Problems	% Mentioning	
	Mothers	Fathers
Specific annoying behaviors	82%	71%
Extramarital affairs	41	41
Serious behavior problems	41	26
Developing in different directions	40	29
Money conflicts	38	38
Child-related conflicts	35	45
Lack of communication	36	32
Irritating personality characteristics	28	36
Physical violence	22	3

When asked to identify the *main reason* for the separation, infidelity and violence were rarely regarded as *primary* (13% of mothers mentioned extra-marital affairs; only 4% mentioned violence; the figures for fathers were 16% and 4%, respectively). The main reason given most often by both mothers and fathers involved behaviors or attitudes one spouse found unacceptable (over 40% of both). Nora Nelson identified Ned's "lack of commitment to married life" as the major cause, mentioning his violence only secondarily. Ned identified Nora's inflexibility as the main problem, as well as her unwillingness to accept him "as a kind, loving person."

For both mothers and fathers, the next most frequently cited main reason was having grown apart (22% of mothers, 16% of fathers). "I think we had different values all along," Christopher Crossland observed. Mothers also fairly often mentioned more severely problematic behaviors, such as alcoholism and gambling (17%, compared with 6 % of fathers).

Although the general difficulties and the main reasons for the separation confirm the impression that broad, longstanding problems in the marriage preceded the decision to separate, it is clear that parents did not always define the difficulties they had experienced in the same terms we might have. For example, it seemed obvious to us that tensions around marital role definitions—often gender based—were problematic for a number of couples. The Elkins, the Stones, and the Crosslands all described serious disagreements about appropriate marital and family roles for husbands and wives. These difficulties were not, however, seen by the couples in these terms (as differences about roles); they were attributed to the personalities or "values" of the partner. We suspect that this attribution difference may result from divorcing individuals' tendency to search for a particular person to blame for the failure of the marriage.

WHERE THE STUDY ENTERED THE STORY:
AFTER THE LEGAL FILING

Near the end of the story of each marriage, parents told us about making the decision to file for divorce. By definition, one of the parents in each family (the mother in 75% of the cases in the mother sample and 56% of the cases in the father sample) had filed for divorce no more than about 6 months prior to talking to us. Filing is a relatively simple act, though it is usually done by lawyers on behalf of clients.

At the time of filing, the individual (or couple) in Massachusetts must specify "grounds" for the divorce. Since 1975, it has been possible to specify "no-fault" grounds (e.g., irretrievable breakdown of the marriage). This approach can be relatively quick, if the two parties are able to file an agreement about custody and division of property at the time of filing. If the couple is *not* able to file an agreement, a no-fault divorce actually takes longer—often twice as long—as a "fault"-based divorce. Therefore, among families in our sample, as in the sampled counties generally, most of the divorces were fault-based. "Cruel and abusive treatment" was the most commonly cited ground (48% of the cases in the mother sample and 36% in the father sample). These grounds usually led to the quickest divorce, but required that the complainant testify to some specific "cruel" or "abusive" behavior. Fewer than one-fifth of the couples were able to file no-fault divorces with agreements about property division and custody, and a third filed for no-fault divorces *without* agreements. In these cases, as well as some of the fault-based cases, a judge must decide on division of property, as well as custody of minor children, if that is in dispute.

As we have seen, initiating the legal process was usually preceded for the adults by a long period of suppressed distress or overt conflict before the actual separation decision. Parents made clear to us that the separation and the legal process were events late in a story that already included a great deal of pain for them—pain they had tried to conceal from their children. Although we will see that many of them talked about feelings of sadness and loneliness after the separation, it is clear that the process of divorce demanded a great deal of active coping effort from them—effort that may have been inconsistent with a prolonged sense of sadness and loss. The demands to address practical and legal issues once the filing had occurred entailed considerable decision making and instrumental activity by the parents.

Across the sample, and regardless of the reasons given for the breakdown of the marriage, by 18 months after the initial separation, the divorces of two-thirds of the mothers and fathers had been finalized or were in the waiting period required before the divorce would be final. Thus, the process of legal divorce was complete within 18 months for most of the couples—in contrast to the processes of both marital dissolution and family transformation, which have much longer courses for most families.

In the course of any divorce, issues of property division, residence, and custody of minor children must be settled. In our families, descriptions of these legal aspects of the divorce—though compelling and critical issues—rarely captured much of the central emotional drama of the divorce. In many cases, decisions were achieved fairly amicably, despite great sadness, distress, and emotional conflict. Parents generally sought to solve the various problems posed by ending their marriage with as little conflict or fallout for the children as they could manage. In only a minority of cases, protracted legal conflict after the separation provided an emotional focus for parents' conflicts (see Johnston, Kline, & Tachann, 1989, for a study of divorces that focuses on custody conflict).

Residence, Custody, and Visitation

Regardless of levels of open family conflict, decisions regarding who would live where were often made with relatively little discussion. In half of the cases, custody and living arrangements were taken for granted (generally the children lived with their mother in the current home). Where there was disagreement, resolutions were based on what seemed best for the children or, less frequently, on practicality. As has been mentioned earlier, almost all the mothers in our study had sole or physical custody of the children at the time of the second interview, and almost half of the participating fathers were awarded sole or physical custody.

Specific visitation schedules were established in about half of the families (this pattern was particularly typical in families where alcohol or violence had been a problem) and left flexible in the others. The typical schedule involved the children spending time with the noncustodial parent (usually the father) every other weekend, often with an additional evening or overnight every week. Sheldon Stone and Ned Nelson each had their children every other weekend, for example, but often called in the middle of the week to arrange a dinner. Eric Elkin's children were with him every Saturday for the full day and every other Sunday (because he had no room for them to sleep over). The Crosslands divided the week into one 3-day and two 2-day units; each took the children for one of the 2-day units each week, and they alternated having them for the 3-day weekend unit.

An impressive two-thirds of the custodial parents reported that they did not find the children's visits with the noncustodial parent stressful, either to arrange or to carry out. However, during the early separation period, about a quarter of the mothers did report that arranging for the visits (establishing where and when the children would be exchanged) was stressful. This was particularly true among the lower income families. Nora Nelson said in the first interview that Ned often "hung around" when he came to get the children, and they would start arguing. When the children came back from these visits it was "hell—the fighting was awful." A year later, slightly *more* mothers (36%) found the visitation arrangements stressful. This was particularly true in families where the father was unemployed or ill, where interparental conflict was high, or where the mother described the child as allied with the father. Visitation was also described as more stressful at the later period by mothers who said their child was angry about the separation. In these cases, visitation may have been stressful because the child was not cooperative about the visits, or it may have been that the mother's perception of the child's negative feelings made her apprehensive about the visitation.

Custody issues were still unresolved at the second time period in 30% of the mothers' cases, with a quarter of these characterized by bitter and intense conflict. This was particularly true where there were boys in the family. In a study of young couples becoming new parents, Cowan and Cowan (1992) also found that, when couples were in conflict, sons were of greater "value" to parents, and daughters were more often ignored or neglected. This probably reflects the greater social value of males generally, as well as cultural beliefs that boys "need fathers" more than girls do. Because divorces usually result in mother-headed households, parents may fear that boys will suffer from father absence more than girls. Twenty-two percent of the fathers reported unresolved custody issues at the later period, with two-thirds of these involving intense conflict (most of the reports of high conflict came from the noncustodial fathers).

Division of Property

By the second interview, agreement regarding property division had been reached by virtually all the couples (90%). The Nelsons were an exception, waiting to hear if the family home would be deeded to Nora, or whether Ned would retain a financial interest (and if so, how much). In any case, despite the fact that most of the mothers in our families retained physical custody of the children, property was described as being equally distributed within the couple according to 45% of the mothers and 30% of the fathers. This was particularly true in families with more resources to begin with; in the case of the Stones, for example, each ended up with a house, a car, and stocks. Somewhat fewer than half of the mothers in both groups were described as having received more property. Fathers were said to have received more by 12% of the mothers and by 25% of the fathers (most in the latter group were custodial fathers).

Forty-seven percent of the mothers and 57% of the fathers said that they and their spouses were both satisfied with the property outcome. About one-third of the mothers and two-fifths of the fathers reported that either they or their ex-spouses were resentful. Given the fact that, on average, mothers experienced a drastic reduction in economic resources as a result of the separation, their low levels of dissatisfaction must be seen as reflecting rather low expectations.

The Legal Process Overall

Half of the mothers and fathers reported that their lawyers were "good" (only a handful of the mothers and none of the fathers said their lawyers were "very good"). Nearly a quarter of the mothers and a third of the fathers felt they were only "okay," and 3% of the mothers and 6% of the fathers felt they were terrible. It is difficult to know how to interpret this lukewarm, but generally positive endorsement of their own attorneys. It does confirm our view that this sample as a whole felt reasonably comfortable with the legal system. Overall, our impression was that these parents, who mostly had racial privilege, some economic or educational resources, and/or confidence in the system, sought to minimize their emotional investment in the legal and financial aspects of the divorce. Their satisfaction may have been due in part to their trust in the legal process. However, it may also have been due to their desire to let go of the marital relationship and to their focus on establishing a new set of family relationships on some stable legal and financial basis. Parents—perhaps especially custodial parents—may literally "settle" for arrangements they think are unfair, out of a strong need to resolve the legal and financial issues.

Most parents wanted to turn to creating a new life and understood this would require giving up aspects of the old one. Concerns about safeguarding the present and future well-being of the children were, for most of the adults, the pervasive and emotionally charged concerns of the postseparation period. As we will see in the next sections, these concerns tended to draw out anxiety about competence and feelings of unmet personal needs more than sadness and loss. Parents sought to establish some sense of order and structure in their lives, but without confidence that they knew what they were doing.

PARENTS' VIEWS OF FAMILY LIFE AFTER THE SEPARATION

Despite the fact that most of the parents were psychologically prepared for the separation, in the sense that they had been thinking about it for a long time, most found life immediately afterward difficult and painful. They struggled both with a new awareness of the losses entailed by the separation and with the high level of demands their new situation, and their children, made on them.

What Changed?

Once the separation had been accomplished, mothers and fathers had to adjust to a new lifestyle, typically one in which they were the only adult in the household. The meaning of this new status differed somewhat, depending on what their household arrangements had previously been (in terms of tasks, how time was spent, etc.) and whether they had custody of the children. It is not surprising that some of the changes were experienced quite differently by mothers and fathers. What is surprising, though, is that in so many instances their experiences were quite similar.

Residence and Finances

Most of the mothers remained in the family house (only 7% moved initially, and another 13% by Time 2). Most of the men moved out (although this was less true of the custodial fathers, 70% of whom remained in the original dwelling, compared to 13% of the noncustodial fathers). As was mentioned in Chapter 2, three-quarters of the mothers were employed outside the home in the initial period following the separation, and they continued or increased their time at work. Nevertheless, consistent with figures reported by other researchers (e.g., Kurz, 1995; Peterson, 1989; Price & McKenry, 1988; Weitzman, 1985, 1988), their financial status deteriorated from what it had been before the separation, with two-thirds saying that their financial situation was worse (half of these said it was much worse).

Household Chores

Prior to the separation, most of the mothers described the division of labor in their families as having followed traditional lines, with the women doing almost all of the daily chores: cooking, dishes, vacuuming, cleaning, shopping, and laundry. About 70% of the mothers reported doing these by themselves, with most of the rest doing them with some help from husbands (16%) and children (9%). Husbands who had helped had primarily contributed to cooking or shopping; they were least likely to be described as helping with cleaning chores. Bill paying had been more evenly split between husbands and wives before the separation. In most households, according to the mothers, the fathers had taken care of yardwork (80%), minor household repairs (75%), and monitoring the family car (85%). (These patterns are quite consistent with those reported by Hochschild, 1989, in her book on working parents.)

The initial impact of the separation was revealed not by the number of daily household chores mothers carried out—they had been doing most of them before and continued to do them—but by the fact that a quarter said their children now helped them. A year later, children were helping with cooking, dishes, and general cleaning in a third of the families (although in fewer than 10% of the families were children ever described as solely responsible for any of these chores). The most noticeable change for mothers was in their taking on the additional chores formerly done by their spouses. After the initial separation, mothers did 90% of the bill paying, 60% of the house repair and car maintenance (the rest of this often shared with a friend or lover), and 44% of the yardwork (the yardwork being shared with children in some of the families). Here, then, mothers were attempting new tasks, but perhaps with considerable anxiety about their ability to handle them. Eventually, though, they took pride in their new skills and abilities, as we shall see below.

Mothers continued to do most of this work a year after the separation. Only about 10% of the mothers had hired help with household chores. At the early time period 40% had child care help, compared with 70% at the later time period, probably reflecting the mothers' increased paid employment. This finding underscores the importance of child care to single mothers, even in this sample of mothers of school-age children. The need would likely be even more dramatic if we had sampled divorcing parents of preschool-age children.

After the separation mothers ended up doing more work in the household, even though they were doing a considerable amount before the separation. The additional tasks were not without some positive aspects, however. For example, Elaine Elkin said that she enjoyed writing "her own checks" ("I've got less money, but at least I decide where it goes now," she said). Nora Nelson commented on how she had "learned a lot of stuff." She added, with some pride, "I can fix a lot of things around the house now."

The fathers' reports of task allotment before and after the separation present a slightly different picture. Most of the fathers described themselves as having been very involved in household chores before the separation. (Obviously either one of the parents is not reporting accurately, or the mother and father samples represent different populations. Because our father sample includes an unusually high percentage of custodial fathers, we suspect the latter.) Half of the custodial fathers said they helped their wives with the traditionally female tasks of cooking, dishes, vacuuming, cleaning, shopping, and laundry (8% indicated they did these tasks without their wives' help). Moreover, two-thirds of the custodial fathers said they had been solely responsible for tasks more stereotypically associated with the male role (i.e., car, house, and yard maintenance), with the rest saying they shared them with their spouses. It may well be that fathers who ended up with custody of their children were indeed those most involved with the household labor before the separation.

Fathers, like mothers, said they performed most of the chores themselves after the separation, with increased help from the children. In about a quarter of both custodial and noncustodial fathers' households, like custodial mothers' households, children helped with cooking, cleaning, and dishes. Custodial fathers were, however, much more likely than either noncustodial fathers or custodial mothers to mention receiving unpaid help from other sources, such as friends, relatives, and ex-spouses, particularly with regard to daily tasks. This willingness of fathers' network members to help with household tasks may be an unexpected benefit of widespread perceptions that men are less experienced or competent than women at household management and child rearing.

For both parents the separation entailed an increase in tasks and chores in the household. This practical aspect of the postseparation period provided a structured pressure for parents actively to cope with their new family situation. This very demand for activity probably encouraged their adaptation, but it was also somewhat incompatible with their own emotional needs. In their accounts of the most difficult parts of their days, parents revealed their sadness, loneliness, and feelings of inadequacy to handle their new situation.

Hardest Part of the Day

When asked to talk about what part of their day seemed the hardest in the early months of the separation, 22% of the mothers and 18% of the fathers said that there was no particular point in the day that was difficult. However, about one-third of the mothers mentioned the times when they were alone, such as after the children were in bed, while about an equal number gave general answers referring to the difficulty of managing their households (e.g., "getting everything done"). Elaine Elkin commented that "having to be with kids all day and cook and clean, get them to bed—there's a lot to do and a lot of confusion." A year later loneliness was less often mentioned as a problem (12%), while managing daily tasks such as getting kids off in the morning (20%) and getting dinner for everyone (25%) seemed harder (compared with 7% and 8% previously).

In general, fathers' responses in the first year focused more exclusively on issues of loss and loneliness (rather than difficulties with coping). More than a quarter mentioned times that reminded them of the loss of the children ("not having them jump in my arms at the end of the day, shouting, 'Daddy,'" as Ned Nelson put it), and 30% mentioned being alone in the evening. Unlike mothers or noncustodial fathers, custodial fathers (20%) also mentioned weekends as being hard (Christopher Crossland complained about weekends when he could never go off and read a book). A year later, fathers mentioned the times when they were alone less frequently (16%); weekends were not mentioned at all. Difficulty at work was mentioned by almost a quarter of the noncustodial fathers, and by 6% of the custodial fathers (compared to 5% and 13% at the initial period) as being the hardest part of the day. None of the mothers mentioned it. Perhaps these men had work difficulties before the divorce. Perhaps, alternately, they found it difficult to concentrate on their work without a supportive home and family context. Finally, it may be custodial parents' life situation that is relevant to understanding this difference. Custodial parents may not see their work lives as a primary context for responding to divorce, because they are so preoccupied with managing their households. In fact, they may see their work as easier to handle than their home life. Nevertheless, bosses and coworkers may notice effects on custodial parents' work lives that those parents may not notice because of their focus on their home lives (see Crosby,1990); noncustodial parents, because they have fewer distractions at home, may be more attentive to problems in the work domain.

Parents' Experiences of Relationships after the Separation

In the sphere of relationships, themes of loss were prominent. Most of the adults regretted the loss of particular aspects of their relationship with their ex-spouse (companionship, help with children, sexual partnership). At the same time, many struggled with questions about how to maintain a parenting relationship with their former partner in the context of their separation. Many adults sought emotional support from friends and relatives and (at widely differing points in the period after the separation) opened themselves to the possibility of establishing new relationships.

Coparenting Relationship

After the separation, most parents maintained some sort of connection with their ex-spouses. This contact varied widely in its nature: an occasional terse phone call to arrange child visits or consult about the legal negotiations; sporadic, but frequent angry calls to express outrage over the settlement being requested or a child care disagreement; regular, business-like communication about the children's activities; weekly visits comparing notes about postseparation life. In a few cases parental visits were warmly companionate and even included overnights during the early period.

   In describing their postseparation relationships in the initial interview, about half of both mothers and fathers reported that their interactions were hostile or tense. This proportion didn't change much over the course of the next year. Time no doubt heals some wounds, but at the 18-month mark, about half of the parents still described their relationship with their ex-spouse as hostile or tense. Both the Nelsons described their relationship as "hostile" at Time 1, and "like a seesaw" at the 18-month mark. Carol Cross-land said their relationship was "meager" at 18 months: "We're really not fond of each other!" On the other hand, one-quarter of the mothers and two-fifths of the fathers described their relationships as "civil" (Sheldon Stone), "pretty decent" (Sheryl Stone), or even mostly "congenial" (Elaine Elkin). These rates are quite similar to those reported in Ahrons (1995) for her sample of men and women experiencing divorce.

Relationships with Friends and Relatives

During the early postseparation period, parents did rely on their friends and relatives to support them and help them through. As Carol Crossland said, "When you go through a trying time and your friends are there for you, you say, 'Wow! They really are the special people I thought they were.' So I value my friends more than ever." At the time of the first interview, 80% of the mothers described themselves as having moderate to frequent contact with close friends (at least once or twice a week, and some even more—Nora Nelson said that in the beginning she might talk to friends on the phone 2 or 3 hours a day). Seventy-five percent described similarly frequent contact with relatives. This high frequency of contact dropped to 70% for friends and 46% for relatives by the time of the second interview, when mothers' needs for social support (and other help) may have been less intense.

Fathers' involvement with friends was a little less frequent, perhaps reflecting a gender difference in the ease with which men talk about personal issues. Ned Nelson said that he didn't see friends too often, other than the two men he lived with, and he certainly didn't talk with them much about the separation ("They don't want to hear about your problems," he commented. "They have enough of their own"). On the other hand, Christopher Crossland talked about "cultivating" friends and being pleased with the progress he'd made in "taking responsibility for making new friends." Overall, though lower than the women's, men's reports of contact with friends were quite high: 60% of the fathers described themselves as having frequent contact with close friends at Time 1 and 55% at the second period. They also maintained relatively high contact with relatives (60% at the first time period and 65% at the second).

It is important to note that a large proportion of both mothers and fathers experienced at least some disapproval from friends and relatives about the divorce. While this should remind us that some sense of stigma was still associated with divorce even in the United States in the 1980s, it may also reflect the tendency of people who feel vulnerable and anxious about what they are doing to be especially attentive to signs of disapproval. Fully 30% of the mothers and 45% of the fathers said they got "some" or "a lot" of disapproval from friends, and even more (about half for both mothers and fathers) mentioned disapproval from some relatives. Christopher Crossland thought part of the problem was that he was the first person in his family of origin to separate from a spouse. Sheldon Stone reported that he rarely saw his widowed father, even though he only lived a town away. "It's too hard to talk to him," he said. "He simply can't understand how things like this can happen." Some disapproval was felt from former in-laws; Carol Crossland, who had been estranged from her own family of origin for some time, felt badly that her ex-spouse's family treated her like she had "ceased to exist." "It's sad," she said, "because I feel like they're my only family I'm close to." On the other hand, Sheryl Stone continued to enjoy a close relationship with her former in-law, who still came to the house on a regular basis to help with child care ("We just don't mention the separation," she said).

Dating

The decrease over time in loneliness noted above in both mothers and fathers may be related to their dating patterns. Although dating frequency was not assessed in the initial period, by the later period only 20% of the mothers were not dating at all, 21% were dating casually, 42% were involved in a serious relationship (most of which include some participation in the daily routines of the household, but not living there), and 16% were living with another partner. Both Carol Crossland and Nora Nelson reported at the second interview that they *had* been involved in serious relationships, but had to break them off; "I don't think I'm ready," Carol commented. The pattern among fathers was similar to the mothers in that only 16% of them were not dating (most of these were custodial fathers). However, of those who were dating, 65% had a steady relationship by the second interview, and 18% were living with someone (as in the case of Mr. Stone). Although some of these relationships may not have been especially good or durable ones, the fact that a substantial proportion of the sample of parents had established a significant intimate relationship within 18 months of the separation suggests that parents were beginning to achieve some adaptation by that time. Moreover, the fact that equivalent numbers of women were dating as men runs counter to the stereotype of divorced women with children having difficulty establishing a social life. At the same time, these results also reflect a clear gender difference, with 83% of the men involved in a steady or committed relationship by the time of the followup and only 58% of the women. This pattern mirrors remarriage rates, which may result from women's recognition of the costs of marriage for them, and men's recognition of its benefits (these have been documented in the literature on mental health and family structure; see Bernard, 1972; Gove, 1978).

Looking Back over the First 18 Months

In the second interview, approximately 18 months after the separation actually took place, mothers and fathers were asked for their overall assessment of what the separation and divorce experience had been like. Looking back over the entire period, both mothers and fathers were most likely to identify the beginning of the process as the worst part, mentioned by 33% of the mothers and 53% of the fathers. Noncustodial fathers were significantly more likely than custodial fathers to identify the beginning as the worst time. (This may have to do with the problems noncustodial fathers had, both in finding and getting settled into new living quarters and establishing a routine with the children. Ned Nelson mentioned, for example, that until he could get his own place he initially stayed with friends. He couldn't "be with the kids the way I wanted to, put them to bed and everything.") Holidays were identified as the worst time by 20% of the mothers, as was the whole process of legal conflict by 27%. Negative contact with their spouse was the worst part for 11% of the mothers, particularly for those with only school-age children (i.e., no preschoolers or adolescents). The legal conflict and lengthy struggle toward a resolution was mentioned by 20% of the fathers, but only a few mentioned holidays (3%) or contact with their spouses (5%).

Parents were also asked about what they saw as the most significant changes in their own lives as a result of the separation experience. Mothers' responses were mostly positive, emphasizing increased happiness, personal growth, self-confidence, and a clearer sense of "self," supporting the notion that divorce can initiate a process of personal growth and development (see, e.g., Bursik, 1991; Stacey, 1990; Riessman, 1990). Nora Nelson said, for example, "It [the separation] made me a lot stronger. I'm getting to really like myself. I guess before I really didn't. I still have my problems, but I can handle them a lot better." Elaine Elkin observed, "It [the separation] made me more independent, made me feel good about myself. Now I do things for myself that I'd never do if I was still married. I go places and I try things. I feel a lot happier now that I don't have all this strain of worrying about what [my husband] wanted me to do." Similarly, Carol Crossland commented, "Overall I'm a happier person; I feel like I'm more myself. I think I had a tendency to be what my husband wanted me to be."

In the sample as a whole, 70% of the mothers felt their personality had changed for the better; 38% felt they had become more independent, 31% said they were happier, and 17% said they experienced less stress than when they were married. Their scores on our psychological measure of mood states were consistent with their responses to the open-ended question about change, showing a significant reduction in anger, tension, depression, fatigue, and confusion. In addition, they showed significant declines in psychological symptoms and an increase in life satisfaction, while self-esteem remained the same. These results are displayed in Figure 3.1.[2]

Some negative aspects of this period were also noted. Of the women, 17% mentioned the loss of companionship. Sheryl Stone, for example, said, "I miss not having an adult to talk to on a regular basis at night. . . . I miss that part of being married, someone to share things with on a regular basis." Eleven percent said they were experiencing more stress as a result of the separation. Elaine Elkin reported that "the last year . . . was a lot more stressful because I wanted everything to get settled . . . I wanted to know . . . how things are going to be so I could make decisions other than worrying about going to court, or what the schedules going to be like for the kids . . . whether I'm go-

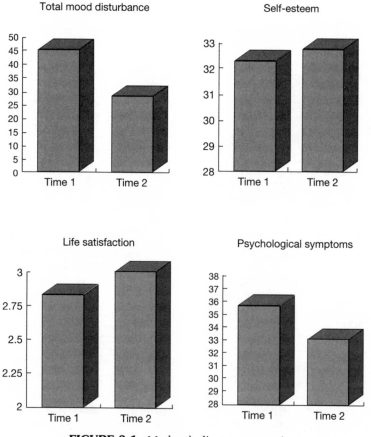

FIGURE 3.1. Mothers' adjustment over time.

ing to work. . . ." Only a few (3%) felt their relationship with their children had worsened, while 11% specifically felt it had improved.

Fathers' responses were also relatively positive: 41% said they were happier and 31% felt their personalities had improved, 25% felt they had become more independent, and 22% said they felt less stress. Better social lives were noted by 18%, and 13% said their relationship with their children had improved. Fathers' scores on our measures of adjustment were consistent with those of the mothers (i.e., negative affect decreased); the statistically significant changes were on anger, confusion, depression, and tension (all of which decreased), life satisfaction (which increased), and the psychological anxiety subscale of the psychological symptoms measure (which decreased). These results are displayed in Figure 3.2.[3]

Nevertheless, fathers' responses about changes focused less than moth-

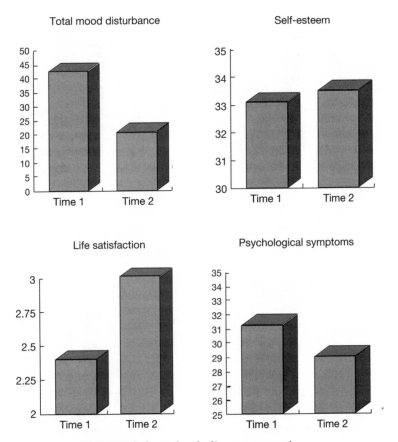

FIGURE 3.2. Fathers' adjustment over time.

ers' on personal growth (e.g., 70% of mothers and 31% of fathers noted positive personality changes). "I feel in more control of my life," said Christopher Crossland. "I'm not in this crazy cycle of guilt where I always felt I could never do enough." "I don't have to argue with my wife anymore," said Ned Nelson, "I don't have all the boiling blood and pounding heart." Sheldon Stone wasn't sure whether the separation had changed his life much at all. "I'm sure things must be different with the children," he answered in response to the question about change, "but I can't tell you what. I'm not sure it's affected me an awful lot." Of the fathers, 19% did say they were lonelier, and a fairly substantial 22% said their relationship with their children had gotten worse (most of the fathers in this category were noncustodial).

THE STRUCTURE OF THE PARENTS' EXPERIENCE

As we pointed out at the outset, there was a pattern to the parents' stories. A painful and protracted period of marital difficulties resulted in a decision to separate and a legal process, which varied widely in the degree of conflict that marked it. After the separation, there was a period in which a sense of loss and helplessness was complicated by many demands for active coping. During the early period after separation, most parents struggled to master their new situation by making efforts to become self-sufficient and competent in handling their new situation. They were focused on these coping efforts and searched for support from others, while showing some continued concerns with loss and sadness. Within 18 months, the weight had shifted toward active coping; a certain degree of emotional equilibrium, perspective, and optimism were clearly in view. These results characterized the early postseparation period more for women than for men. This difference may reflect well-documented gender differences in marriage and family roles, emphasizing men's competence and women's dependence (themes reflected in many of the women's statements). By contrast with the marriage, the postseparation period for women involved an increased household burden, but also a heady sense of release from a confining role and a chance to develop new skills and qualities. Men experienced a similar increase in burdens, and many of the same anxieties about their ability to handle them, but without the same sense of release and opportunity.

By the 18-month mark, however, both men and women were often inclined to adopt the view summed up by one man:

> "Treat it as reality. This is the way it's going to be. The two-parent household isn't the only way to be—this can be okay too. If you spend time saying, 'Oh, gee, this could have been like this, and that could have been like that,' you miss out on what's really there now. And so do your kids."

Embedded in the parents' accounts, then, we find two stories: the end of a marriage, in which separation and divorce is the climax and gendered marital roles are a key background; and the transformation of a family structure, in which separation and divorce is the beginning. Seen this way, the complexity of parents' emotional experience of divorce is easy to understand. This perspective also helps explain the significant differences in how parents and children experience separation and divorce. For children, separation and divorce were the shocking beginning of the story—one with no happy ending in sight, at least at first. One useful way to formulate the differences in parents' and children's experience may be in terms of a general theory about the psychological process of adaptation to life changes.

ADAPTING TO LIFE CHANGES

In an attempt to integrate a variety of findings about responses to different kinds of life changes, Stewart (1982) proposed a general account of the emotional process of adaptation to changed external circumstances. She suggested that when individuals face any situation that involves dramatic and pervasive change in their lives (a new school or job, a new country, a new marital or family situation), they adopt a series of psychological stances toward their external environment. Thus, marked changes in life circumstances bring about a marked change in psychological orientation. Normally, when we are in familiar surroundings, the environment simply provides a background for our actions. When we are in a new situation, we are much more self-conscious and at the same time more attentive to the environment.

In thinking about parental separation and divorce in these terms, we must notice that the first big changes for many parents were really not changes in the environment as much as changes inside themselves—changes in their feelings, hopes, and wishes. Although there were certainly changes in their relationships, many parents let us know that many of those changes had happened long before there was any thought of separation. Sheryl Stone said:

> "I think in a way there was a certain amount of my withdrawing 6 years ago . . . not consciously, really. But when I decided to go back to school, Sheldon was not at all supportive. . . . He wasn't supportive of me in a way that I felt I needed. My taking myself in a totally new direction when I went back to school was one of the first times when I really picked myself up and made a decision that was for me. That was the first step. And then that gave me more freedom to totally make my own decisions after that."

Later, for many divorcing parents there were changes in the environment—changes in the household for parents who lived with their children, changes in residence for parents who did not, and often job and social life changes for all of them. It may be that in the case of divorce the reorientation process is signalled at very different points, depending on the individual's experience of change. For some it may come with a serious disappointment in the marriage; for others it may be the news of a partner's dissatisfaction (Sheldon Stone described himself as "stunned"); or it may even happen when a partner moves out, or after a move to a new apartment and a single life.

In a series of studies Stewart and her colleagues (Stewart, Sokol, Healy, Chester, & Weinstock-Savoy, 1982; Stewart, Sokol, Healy, & Chester, 1986; Stewart & Healy, 1985, 1992) showed that in the initial period following a major life change, people adopt a broadly *passive and receptive* stance toward the external environment. This stance (like the subsequent ones; see Table 3.2 for an illustration of the four stances) is reflected in four domains: feelings; and orientations toward action, authority figures, and friends and loved ones. When people are in new and unfamiliar situations, they tend to be relatively *passive* and to avoid taking actions, perhaps quite sensibly because they have little understanding of the likely implications of actions. For our divorcing parents, this passivity may be reflected in difficulties getting around to filing

TABLE 3.2. Thematic Concerns Defining Four Stances toward the Environment Following a Major Life Change

Stance	Attitude toward authority	Relations with others	Feelings	Orientation to action
Receptive	Authorities are benevolent; they help, advise, praise	Others will fulfill one's wishes and meet needs	Feelings of sadness, loss, and confusion	Passivity and inaction
Autonomous	Authorities are critical and punitive, concerned with rules, not people	Others will *not* fulfill wishes or meet needs	Anxiety about competence; indecision	Action to protect self from intrusion; limited, reactive to situations
Assertive	Opposition to authority; view of authority as corrupt	Others as objects to use and exploit; no mutuality	Anger and hostility to others	Confident initiative but failure due to errors in judgment
Integrated	Authorities seen as "human," with limited power and constraints	Others as differentiated from self and full partners in relations	Complex, ambivalent feelings toward others	Commitment to and emotional involvement in work

for separation or finding a new apartment, once the decision to separate has been made. After changes, people are also likely to experience *feelings of loss and sadness* over the fact that they have given up the more familiar (even if undesirable) previous situation. Thus, even while people happily embrace some life changes, they often also experience a sad awareness of what they have left behind (see, e.g., Weiss, 1975). This feature of the receptive stance was clearly reflected in most of the divorcing parents' stories; it was part of both the story of the end of their marriage and the story of their new beginning in a new family structure.

Immediately after life changes, people tend to focus on *having their own needs met* in their orientation toward other people, including from authority figures. Some of this tendency may have been reflected in many parents' search for emotional support from friends and relatives and in their lack of enthusiasm for their lawyers. Thus, some features of the receptive stance clearly characterized the divorcing parents' experience, but this stance was present both before and after the separation, and for different people it may have predominated at different points in the process.

For most parents, whether they were living with or away from their children, many external demands pulled them away from a receptive stance. In their studies of the course of adaptation to new situations, Stewart and her collegues demonstrated that, over time, individuals adopted more active stances. Although parents may have adopted the passive, receptive stance when they first recognized their marriage could not continue, at least once the filing took place, all of them had many things they needed to do to create and maintain a new family structure. Parental separation may differ importantly from other life changes adults experience—new jobs, getting married, bereavement, perhaps even divorce without children—in leaving little room for passivity, reliance on benevolent authorities, awareness of loss and sadness, and a focus on getting one's own needs met after the change itself. The demands to address practical and legal issues, as well as children's emotional needs, may draw parents rather quickly into the anxious indecision, or even the hostile confrontation, of the next two stances.[4]

In contrast to the receptive stance, a coherent *autonomous* stance did characterize many parents' accounts of the period immediately following parental separation. In this stance, the individual begins to attempt to take action, but focuses on relatively narrow *efforts to create order* in what feels like a chaotic situation (Elaine Elkin's pleasure at being able to "write her own checks" and Nora Nelson's at being able to "fix a lot of things around the house" are good examples of this kind of orientation to action). Often these efforts are accompanied by *feelings of uncertainty and indecision,* and relations with others (including authorities) are focused on a sense of *others' failures to be helpful or supportive enough.* Clearly many of the feelings the parents reported at the first interview—particularly their concerns about other people's disapproval of their actions and their worries about whether they could handle the situation—fit this description.

The third stance associated with life changes involves more vigorous *self-assertion*, with the individual *risking failure by bold actions*. Perhaps because the dominant emotion is *hostility*, relations with others tend to be *conflictual or exploitative*, and *authority figures are seen as corrupt and exploitative* too. This assertive, sometimes hostile stance was reflected in some individuals' relations with their former partners even at the first interview. Throughout the postseparation period, efforts to pursue new relationships, new jobs or promotions, and more education reflected a willingness to take risks. Somewhat negative or cynical views of the legal system and resentment of others' disapproval reflected other aspects of this stance.

By the second interview, 18 months after the separation, many parents seemed to have moved well beyond the autonomous stance, and some had moved beyond the assertive stance as well. When the individual has really adapted to a new situation, an *integrated* stance is adopted. Here the individual is capable of *effective work commitments*, can tolerate *ambivalent feelings*, can accept *authority figures as limited in their power*, and can establish *fully mutual relationships with others*. Within 18 months of parental separation, it is perhaps too much to expect people to attain a fully integrated stance, but we did see some evidence of increased tolerance of ambivalence, realistic appreciation of the new situation, and growth in a capacity for mutual relationships. The fact that many of the parents—especially the mothers—reported a sense of real personal growth as a result of the divorce may be significant and may relate directly both to eventual movement toward an integrated stance, and to the overall sequence of stances.

Stewart has argued that the process of adapting to new situations, especially because of the openness to influence characteristic of the receptive stance, provides adults with new opportunities for personality change and growth. Stewart and Healy (1985) showed that college students who retained the receptive stance during their first year showed more substantial gains in critical thinking during the course of their college experience. In related research, Bursik (1986) found that divorcing women showed more personality growth in terms of ego development, if they had adopted the receptive stance. Thus, although the receptive stance often feels embarrassingly childish and unpleasant to adults in our culture, it does seem to permit adults the very advantages of childhood: the opportunity to develop and change.

Thinking about the parents' overall process of adaptation to separation and divorce can help us understand how profoundly "out of synch" parents and children in our families were bound to be in their early responses to the actual separation. In the next chapter we will see that 6 months after their parents' separation, when their parents were mostly focused on issues of autonomy or even assertiveness, the children in our families were struggling—

as the theory led us to expect—with a painful, receptive stance toward their new family situation.

NOTES

1. Because we were focusing on the process of change over time in this chapter, responses are drawn from the core longitudinal sample of 103 mothers and 34 fathers who participated with their children over the entire 18-month period of the study. Custodial and noncustodial fathers' responses are presented as a single group, except where their experiences were different enough to warrant reporting them separately. Responses were coded into the categories described in the text; many parents mentioned more than one kind of problem, so we report the percentage of all parents reporting each kind of problem. In all of the analyses in this chapter, we considered whether gender, custody, or family characteristics—religion, family size, socioeconomic status—made a difference in the divorce experience. Except for gender and custody, they mostly did not. Where there were gender or custody (or, rarely, other) differences in patterns, they are discussed in the text.

   Throughout this chapter material from the interview is described. Verbatim transcripts of the interviews were coded, with first- and second-year interviews mixed together, for themes discussed here and throughout this book. Coders achieved interrater agreement on the presence of themes above .85 (using the percent agreement formula for content analysis discussed in Smith, 1992) and reliability at this level was maintained by systematic double coding and spot checking.

2. Repeated-measures analyses of variance ($df = 1,97$) indicated over-time changes for mothers that were significant for mood disturbance, anger–hostility, confusion–bewilderment, depression–dejection, tension–anxiety, and fatigue–inertia, as well as for life satisfaction and psychological symptoms, $p < .05$. There was no change on self-esteem. Means are displayed in Appendix Table 3.1.

3. Repeated-measures analyses of variance ($df = 1,33$) indicated that scores for fathers on total mood disturbance, anger–hostility, confusion–bewilderment, depression–dejection, tension–anxiety, life satisfaction, and the psychological anxiety subscale of the symptoms measure reflected significant over-time change, $p < .05$. There were no changes on fatigue–inertia, vigor–activity, self-esteem, overall psychological symptoms, or the illness and immobilization subscales of psychological symptoms. Means are displayed in Appendix Table 3.2.

4. Another possibility, which we cannot fully rule out, is that divorcing parents who *did* retain the receptive stance after separation did not participate in the study, because they lacked the energy or will to do so. Given the overall representativeness of the sample, this seems unlikely.

CHAPTER 4

The Children's Stories

Many of the children in our study learned about their parents' separation at a kind of informal family "press conference," at which the news was announced. Some of the children's accounts were pretty matter of fact. One 7-year-old told us, "One day they sat down and talked to me and my brother about it. That's how I knew." An 8-year-old boy described the announcement in his family somewhat more vividly:

> "One night, they had a big fight. We [the three children] were playing [a computer game]. So we went to our room 'cause we thought maybe we should leave them alone. Then, my father came in. He said—he approached it gently—and then he finally came out with 'We're getting divorced.' And that's how we knew."

Some children had hazier memories, but they nevertheless recalled simply "being told" that their parents were separating. For example, a 14-year-old boy told us, "I guess my mother told me—I don't know. One of them told me." Despite the vagueness of his reply, he did recall that his mother told him, "They weren't getting along and he's going to move out for a little while," and his father told him, "When you're older, I'll tell you the whole story." This boy remembered his own responses very clearly indeed: "I was pretty sad. I might have cried a little. I was pretty mad at my father for leaving, though. He hadn't been coming home much anyway."

Although many of the children, like that boy, were aware of their parents' fights or absences, they rarely *expected* a divorce and still experienced the news of the separation as shocking. One 6-year-old girl told us that her

This chapter was drafted by Nia Lane Chester and Abigail J. Stewart.

mother told her and her brother that she and her father were separating "'cause they don't love each other anymore." Although she was surprised by this news, she also told us this:

> "When they were going to fight, I said, 'Stop it!' I'd say, 'Stop it' 'cause when I was trying to get to bed I would hear *all* of it. There was lots of sounds and I could hear it. I couldn't get to sleep. That was a long time ago. . . ."

She did not view the conflict as either escalating or signalling a likely family transformation. Instead, she saw it as a persistent, though unpleasant feature of her family life.

Some children were not really told directly that their parents were separating. One child was told by his friend:

> "My mom told my friend, but my friend told me. She told my friend not to tell me 'cept he told me because he thought I should know about my mom and dad getting divorced. I said, 'Are you kidding?' He said, 'No.' I said, 'You'd better be telling the truth.' And so then I found out that he was telling the truth."

He found this out as his parents gradually informed him of what was going on (first telling him they didn't get along, then that they were going to live apart for awhile, then that they were getting divorced). As he described it, "They were telling it to me the easy way, not the hard way, like I'd get upset all at once. Then they told me about some of it each day." He never told them that he had already heard the news from his friend, "'cause I didn't want them to think that my friend wasn't a good secret keeper."

Although fairly unusual, quite a few children were either told the day of the separation or simply witnessed their parent's departure or absence. A 9-year-old told us that his whole family was at home and his father "called us down and he told us that they were getting separated." The father said, "Since your mom and I aren't getting along good, it's come to an end and we have to get a separation." Then his father left. In another family a 10-year-old told us he learned about the separation as it happened. He and his sister "were watching TV in the other room. They were in the kitchen arguing. My mother told him to leave the house." No real "announcement" was made; his parents' actions spoke for themselves. And in subsequent weeks his parents did talk about it with him.

Children's stories about their parents' separations and divorces were, then, quite different from their parents'. They were stories with sudden, often dramatic beginnings. They were most typically stories of the unexpected announcement or discovery of bad news, followed by accounts of how they and their families coped both with the news and their new situations. These accounts, unlike their parents', did not—could not—focus on the legal and practical issues involved in creating separate households. They do not include descriptions of plans made or actions taken. Instead, the children described a situation changing around them that they had little ability to control. While the parents' stories emphasize decisions and instrumental efforts, the children's focus on reactions—things to be glad about, to be mad about, to resent, or to miss. In this way, the children and the parents had very different stories to tell about their experience.

WHOSE STORY ABOUT CHILDREN'S EXPERIENCE SHOULD WE BELIEVE?

In planning how to assess children's experience of their parents' separation and divorce, we wondered who was the best source of information—a parent or the child? In many psychological studies, researchers assume that children cannot report directly on their experience (or at least cannot do so very well); therefore, parents (and sometimes teachers) are often used as informants about children's responses to events. While recognizing that all people—adults and children—are unaware of some of their motivations, feelings, and impulses, we proceeded on the assumption that it was worthwhile to listen directly to what children had to say, and to take it seriously. It seemed to us that considerable harm has been done to powerless people—among them children—when psychologists have simply assumed that it was not reasonable to take what they said seriously (see, e.g., the debate among psychoanalysts about whether to "believe" young women's accounts of the unwelcome sexual advances of older men, including their fathers; as well as the discussion of whether to believe children's accounts of sexual abuse both in psychology and the law). Moreover, and most importantly, we suspected that children would have valuable things to say about their own experience—perhaps things that parents and teachers would not know. There were cases, for example, where children protected their parents from knowledge, like the child who did not let his mother know that his friend had already told him about the separation.

In other instances, parents may have been so caught up in painful events that they didn't process how much their children knew about what was going on. For example, one mother told us that her 8-year-old daughter learned about the separation "the day after the fight. . . . He was gone and she knew that I wanted him out of there. . . . I didn't hide it from her." In contrast, the child told us that she found out this way:

> "I heard the fight. And then the next morning everything was all a mess—broken. And I got up in the middle of the night, and there was a

steak in the chair. My father threw a steak at my mother. We usually go across the neighbors when my parents get in a fight—when my father locks my mother out of the house, and my mother tries to break in. When she found out she was locked out, she went in the back door. But I didn't go over there now because the police took him away. My mother called the police and they said, 'If you do anything wrong we're going to have to put you in jail.' So she had to call again because he did it again—so they took him. . . . That was the night, that was what did it. I hated it when he had to leave, because I had to pack all the clothes."

This child's memories of witnessing the fight and the police coming, and of packing her father's clothes were important parts of her experience of her parents' separation. These aspects of the child's experience were not reported, perhaps not recognized, by her mother, who no doubt wished she had been able to protect her child from this terrible scene.

We found that many children, even very young ones, were able to tell us about what happened and how they felt about it. For example, one second grader told us about how her parents told her about their separation:

"(*Do you know why your parents decided not to live together anymore?*) Yes. Because they can't get along together and they'll be much happier when they're separated so they won't fight as much. (*How did you find out about it?*) My mother told me. (*How?*) She said, 'Paula, Elaine, me and your father are getting a divorce.' She just told me. My mother never lies. My sister might [lie] a little bit. My father doesn't lie to me either. (*What did your dad say?*) Well, my mother kicked him out before he could say anything. (*Did you talk about it with him later?*) Yeah, plenty of times. He says, 'You know, Elaine, we're getting a divorce because me and your mother can't handle, we can't stay together 'cause we're gonna fight all the time. That's why we're getting a separation.' (*How did you feel when they told you?*) Well, pretty sad, but I got used to it after awhile."

Like many of the children quoted in this chapter, Elaine had definite memories about what had happened, and she was able and willing to tell us about them, and about her feelings. At the same time, partly because we were aware that the children in the study might not be able to articulate their experience well (especially the youngest), and partly because it is always helpful to have multiple perspectives, we assumed that information about the children from their parents would be valuable. Therefore, in this chapter we will describe reports of both the "focus children" and their mothers. In general, the pattern of responses did not depend on the gender or age of the child (within the study age limits, children were between 6 and 12 years old); when there were differences between older and younger children, or between boys and girls, we will mention it. As we have seen, although there is overlap in the accounts by mothers and their children, there are also differences; these differences do not suggest to us that either reporter was "better." Instead, they tend to reveal differences in the parents' and children's perspectives. These differences arise not only because of parents' wishes to present children with reasonable decisions rather than violent scenes, but also because parents are aware of certain details children may not notice.[1]

We can compare two accounts of how children were first told about the impending separation. These excerpts are taken from interviews with members of the Stone family described in Chapter 3; we will refer to all four of the the families described in that chapter at various points in this one. Recall that the Stones' separation had resulted from Sheryl's gradual alienation from Sheldon and the marriage. Here's how their 9-year-old daughter, Sally, learned about it:

> "First my mother started to tell us but then my father said, 'She'll probably never get to tell you,' so he told us that they're gonna get divorced. My mother was kind of sad about it, so she kept pausing, so finally my father told us instead. (*How did you feel about it when they told you?*) Sad. (*Do you know why your mom and dad decided not to live together any more?*) They said they were having lots of arguments. So they weren't going to live together, and they were getting divorced."

Sheryl recalls the same scene this way:

> "We brought the kids into the family room, and I was going to tell them, but I burst into tears. So their father proceeded to tell them what we had agreed to tell them—that we have been having arguments, that were not about kids, but that they didn't know [about the arguments] because we had the arguments after they were in bed; that we felt that we would be a lot happier if we were not living together, and that's what we were going to do; and that their father was going to move out the next week—he would have a separate house, and they would get to see him there.(*How did the children react?*) Sam looked very sad, but did not cry. Sally cried, and she cried a lot. And Sandra sucked her thumb for a while. Then the thumb comes out of her mouth, and she says, 'I know somebody whose parents are divorced. There're lots worse things than having your parents get divorced!'"

Although clearly Sheryl's account has more details, especially details about what the parents said, and how the other children reacted, Sally's own account conveys her experience pretty clearly.

In contrast to most of the parents, we have seen that children heard about the impending separation as "news" about a consequential and unwelcome event that was—though not accomplished—inevitable. A little over half of the mothers reported that their children learned about the separation from them (30%), from both parents (17%), or from their fathers (9%), shortly before a parent (usually the father) had actually moved out. However, they reported that over one-quarter of the children didn't find out about the separation until it was occurring. This was more common in families where the father's behavior had included violence or substance abuse. They described the remaining children in our sample (17%) as having figured it out for themselves (this was more common among older children).

Overall, children's reports suggested a slightly higher rate of parental informing: 68% said they were told by one or both parents before the actual separation, and 30% said they learned during or after the separation. This kind of discrepancy probably arises from parents and children identifying different moments as when children were "told." For example, in the first section of this chapter we heard a 10-year-old boy's account that he and his brother overheard his mother ask his father to leave. His mother described the same story, but said that she had not really talked with the children at that point. She said, "I found it a difficult subject to approach with them." Instead, over a period of weeks she said she put questions to them: "I find that the situation is very difficult to live with—how do you feel about it? I find that Dad's behavior is unacceptable—how do you feel about it in your life?" After asking these questions for awhile, during a visit to her parents over the holidays she said to the boys, "You've heard me ask your father to leave. Is that acceptable to you—don't go home until he's gone? They both said yes." Thus, from her perspective she really didn't tell them about the separation at all. They joined with her in making the decision. But from the child's perspective, once he heard his mother tell his father to leave, he had heard the news.

What the mothers said they told the children was relatively consistent with what the children remember being told. Almost half (44%) of the mothers said they told the children they were separating because they couldn't get along and were always fighting (as the Stones did). In fact, in the case of the Stones, fighting had not been a particularly prominent feature of the marital problems before the separation. But "fighting" was something they thought the children could understand.

Parents were somewhat less likely to admit to the children that the reason had to do with problematic behavior of one of the parents, unless it was fairly extreme, and probably also visible to the child, such as alcoholism or mental illness. Thus, although 43% of the mothers had mentioned unacceptable behaviors to the interviewer as the main reason for the separation, and 13% had indicated affairs, these reasons were given to the children at rates of only 10% and 2%, respectively. This difference probably reflects the mothers' assumption that it would be best for children if they did not describe the separation in terms that seemed to blame the other parent. It may also reflect their efforts to put the explanation into a form they felt the child/ren could understand (by describing symptoms to the children, rather than what mothers perceived to be the underlying cause). Thus, Sheryl Stone told us that the separation had resulted from her husband's unwillingness to support her development, but her husband told the children that it was because "we had been having arguments, that they were not about the kids, but that they didn't know because we had the arguments after they were in bed." The fact that parents and children often had different understandings of the reasons for the separation provides one more basis for continuing differences in their experience of the family transformation.

Mothers were more likely to be consistent in giving children explanations for the divorce in cases where extreme behavior (alcoholism, gambling, etc.) was involved; about 20% of the mothers gave such an explanation to both the interviewer and their children. Very few of the mothers (2%) mentioned physical violence to the children as a reason for the divorce (including Nora Nelson, who only referred to Ned's drinking). Perhaps partly because the separation period was chaotic and stressful, 16% of the mothers said they didn't recall what they told the children. It may be that they actually did not tell the children anything, because over a quarter of the children (disproportionately the younger ones) said they were not given any explanation of the separation at all.

Most parents (90%) assumed that their children understood most or all of what they had been told, and in fact the children were able to reproduce the reasons they were told. Thus, two-thirds of the children told the interviewer their parents were separating because they were always fighting and/or couldn't get along. While some children gave only short explanations (from Sally Stone: "They were having lots of arguments"), others were more complicated (from one of the Crossland children: "They were fighting a lot. My dad always went to work and my mom took care of us; my father cooked and stuff, but he didn't do as much as my mom and she goes to school too, and she had to do too much. There's a million more reasons, that's just one. I can't remember the others right now").

Another 17% of the children mentioned specific negative behaviors of one of the parents (e.g., "Dad was never home"), while a relatively large proportion (28%) mentioned serious behavior problems (e.g., Nancy Nelson simply said the reason was "because my dad drinks"). Less then 1% mentioned physical violence or loving someone else.

Overall, the process of "breaking the news" to the children was recalled fairly vividly by both children and parents; they often recalled and described the time of day, the place, where each family member was, and what was said and done. From research on "flashbulb" and "vivid" memories, we know that events recalled like this tend to be ones that are novel or unexpected, emotionally charged, and viewed by the person as likely to be consequential (see Brown & Kulik, 1977; Pillemer, Rhinehart, & White, 1986; Rubin, 1986). The very fact that in these memories parents were informants and children were passive recipients of information underlines how the parents' role demanded something different from the passivity of the receptive stance at the precise moment it was being elicited in the children.

CHILDREN'S INITIAL REACTIONS TO THE NEWS

About half the children, according to parents, reacted with visible distress and tears to the news of the separation, but they tended not to object or ask questions in response. A few parents (9%) described the children as angry or protesting (as in the case of Carl Crossland, who "stamped his foot and shouted, 'No, you're *not!*'") A similar number (8%) said their children responded by asking for information ("Where will Daddy live?" "Where will I live?"), and a surprising number (18%) had no visible reaction, according to the parents. Finally, a few children (8%) were described as apparently relieved.

Parents were also asked to talk about what they perceived their children's feelings about the separation to be, regardless of what the child actually said or did. Parents' responses confirmed an overall impression that the children experienced the news as about an important and painful loss. Of the mothers, 37% said their children were generally "upset." This response was particularly likely in lower-income families and less common in families where the father had been alcoholic or violent. Most of the remaining parents mentioned a range of more specific negative emotions, listed in Table 4.1. On the other hand, 15% of the children were described as feeling relieved, particularly in families where the father had been alcoholic or violent (e.g., both Mr.

TABLE 4.1. Children's Feelings about Their Parents' Separation

Feeling	% Reported spontaneously by	
	Mother	Child
Upset; generally bad	37%	30%
Sad	18	54
Scared; surprised	10	8
Confused	14	3
Angry	14	8
Rejected	3	0
Guilty	2	<1
Relieved	15	10

and Ms. Nelson thought Nancy found it easier without all the fighting going on).

The children themselves were asked how they felt when they heard about or learned that their parents were going to separate. This question was posed first in an open-ended way. Later in the interview children were asked whether they now felt a particular way "a lot, a little, or not at all." When asked the open-ended question about how they felt at the time that they were told, children's answers were consistent with their parents' perceptions, at least in the sense of feeling bad and focusing on feelings of loss: more than half said they felt sad (as Sally Stone had), and another third gave vague negative answers ("bad," "terrible," "not good"). A few said they felt angry, surprised, or confused. About one-tenth said they felt glad or relieved. Only one child mentioned feeling like it was his fault in response to the open-ended question (Table 4.1 includes these figures).

When children were asked about specific emotions they might feel "about their parents' separation" (with no particular time referent), they revealed a wider range of feelings (see Table 4.2 for exact percentages). While by far the dominant emotion was sadness, more than half said they felt confused, scared, or surprised. Although few parents thought the children felt guilty, and many said they specifically told the children not to blame themselves, about a third of the children agreed they felt "like it was partly my fault" (though only a handful said they felt this a lot). It is not clear whether children felt guilty in spite of their parents' reassurances, or whether their parents' frequent protestations to the contrary made them feel that perhaps they *were* responsible in some way! Certainly a number of parents (about one-third) implicated child-rearing issues as a source of tension in the family, which may have been internalized by children as their responsibility. The Elkins' daughter, for example, probably witnessed her parents' arguments

TABLE 4.2. Children's Responses to Questions about Particular Feelings

Feelings	% Children responding at Time 1 that they feel that way	
	A lot	A little
Sad	50%	32%
Confused	22	34
Scared	22	34
Surprised	15	27
Like it's partly my fault	4	31
Angry	13	33
Glad	11	20

about whether she should be allowed to play at other people's houses. Children were also more likely to acknowledge feeling angry in response to the specific question, with a third saying they felt this way a little, and 13% saying they felt angry a lot.[2]

Perhaps children were less likely to bring up anger or guilt on their own because they thought they should not feel them, or perhaps they were less salient or dominant feelings than sadness, and therefore overshadowed by it. For example, the 8-year-old boy whose parents told the children about the separation while they were playing a computer game described his reaction as feeling "sad." He also said, in response to the closed-ended questions that he felt "a lot" sad, "a little" angry, and "a little" scared. Some clues to his anger are contained in his extended discussion of the reasons his parents separated (as opposed to what they told him, which was that they fought too much). He said:

> "My mother really didn't care for my father because he took the wedding ring off, and so she didn't like the way that happened. She thinks he cheats on her—I don't know much about that."

Thus, although the "official story" is about fighting, this child knows something about the background of that story, which makes him angry and scared, as well as sad.

The overall impression from mothers and children was that children responded to the news of their parents' separation with feelings of sadness and loss, as well as confusion and fear—defining features of the receptive stance. As one first grader put it:

> "My mother told me and I was shocked. And I was scared. I was crying for 2 days, and I was sad. I thought my father wasn't gonna be my father any more."

Like most of the children, this boy felt he was in a passive role (recipient of news) and was helpless to change the situation, though he did not like it.

At the time of the second interview, the intensity of children's negative feelings had lessened somewhat in the responses to the inquiries about specific emotions. For example, only 20% (compared to 32%) said they still felt sad "a lot," and 28% (compared to 18%) said they didn't feel sad at all. Eighty percent said they did not feel at all guilty (compared to 65% at the time of the separation). Nevertheless, the level of anger remained about the same (with 30% still feeling "a little" angry and 9% feeling angry "a lot"), as did the feelings of being scared and confused (still felt at least a little by about half the sample). The open-ended answers tended to mirror a greater acceptance of the divorce, at least among the older children. "I figure it was their decision, so I don't mind or anything," commented Sam Stone. Nancy Nelson commented, "I don't care. I wouldn't want him to come back. It's better now." Of course some of their answers probably reflect some denial, as we hear more directly in Carl Crossland's remark at the second interview:

> "I don't have any feelings about it anymore. (*Do you remember what you used to feel?*) No, I don't remember. I don't have feelings." [He answered "not at all" to all the closed-ended items about specific emotions.]

Overall, the receptive stance was receding at the second interview, but it was still partially present. This persistence indicates that the separation posed a major adaptive challenge to the children; it was hard for them to move on. It is probably also due to children's relatively passive role in the situation of parental divorce, as well as the fact that the postseparation period generated additional changes in their lives. These changes—equally imposed from outside—may have required adaptation and adjustment too.

For example, during the postseparation period, almost 40% of the children admitted to having felt caught in loyalty conflicts between their parents at some point. These feelings resulted from a variety of situations, some of which seemed relatively unavoidable. One girl explained that her Dad's girlfriend let them make a special meal at his house, and when she described it to her mother, asking if they could recreate it in the mother's kitchen, the girl felt the mother "maybe got a little jealous and I felt bad I'd talked about it." Other situations seemed a lot more direct on the part of a parent. For example, another girl said that whenever "I'm talking to Dad and I say 'our' TV or 'our' house, he gets mad and says, 'It's *my* TV and *my* house! Your mother thinks she's getting everything but she's not!'" The need to address these issues, as well as many others (new people in their lives, changed schools or residences, etc.) may well serve to prolong children's adaptation to parental separation.

CHILDREN'S REACTIONS AFTER THE SEPARATION

Like the children's divorce-related feelings, both the children's psychological adjustment and their behavior (as indicated by the psychological tests they took both years, and the parent and teacher reports) were significantly improved at Time 2, compared with Time 1.[3] There was no change on reports of children's physical illness (see Figure 4.1 and Appendix Table 4.1). In Chapter 6 we will see that it is unlikely that this improvement is the result of children simply getting older, because older and younger children did not differ in adjustment within each time period. Instead, the improvement in self, mother, and teacher perceptions probably results from the passage of time since the separation.

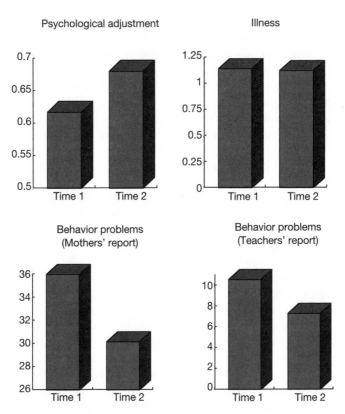

FIGURE 4.1. Children's adjustment over time.

Parents' interview accounts were consistent with these data. For example, parents indicated that about 20% of the children talked about the separation a lot in the initial period, but half as many were still doing so a year later. Girls were more likely to talk about it at both times, as were children whose parents' own parents had been divorced. The topics most of the children focused on were the possibilities of reconciliation (15% at both time periods) and remarriage to someone else (20% at the early period and 24% a year later). Older children were more likely to talk about remarriage at the initial separation period, while younger children were more likely to talk about it at the later period (when perhaps the possibility was more obvious). When parents were asked directly whether they thought their children hoped for a reconciliation, 26% said yes at the initial period, but only 14% at the later period. (Carol Crossland said in the second interview that Carl had recently asked, "When are you two going to get together again?" "I had no idea he was still thinking that," she said.) Another third said that their children gave signs of wanting a reconciliation in the first few months, even though they didn't express this desire directly. In general, though, it seems that children and their parents did not talk about the separation or divorce very much. (This impression is confirmed by the fact that so many parents mentioned that a benefit of participating in the study was that they had a good talk with their children about the divorce; see Chapter 2.)

When asked about what they thought was the hardest thing for the child to get used to in the whole process, loss themes were prominent in parents' accounts. Forty-four percent of the mothers mentioned the absence of the father (particularly often mentioned when there were boys in the family), 20% said the fact of the separation itself, and the rest mentioned other divorce-related changes, such as school changes, less money, and residence changes (the latter being mentioned more often by mothers of girls).

Similarly, themes of loss predominated in children's answers to the question about what they thought was worse about their lives since the separation. One-third identified not having their father in the house as the hardest thing, or having to see each parent "one at a time." The separation itself was mentioned by 9% (Sally Stone said, "I don't see either of them as much as I used to"), and a handful (3% each) mentioned having less money and other resources, or more rules and responsibilities. Still, over a third said that nothing was worse. Given that two-thirds of the mothers felt their financial situations were worse, it is interesting that so few of the children identified having less money or fewer resources as a problem.

Children also talked about what seemed better after the separation. Although a third couldn't think of anything that was better, over a quarter identified the absence of conflict between their parents. Fewer problems because of the father being gone was mentioned by 13% of the children, as was having more resources available (16%). A few children (7%) also mentioned getting to see their father more as a benefit of the separation. "I never saw my dad before much except sometimes on weekends. Now when I'm with him, I'm with him the whole weekend," one of the Stone children commented. In striking contrast to the parents' accounts, children's accounts of positive and negative postseparation changes in the household focused on the absence of the non-custodial parent and the diminution of conflict, rather than an increase in tasks and responsibilities in the family.

Mothers were asked to assess the effects of the separation or divorce on specific areas of the child's life. With regard to school, half did not see any effect at either time period. About 14% said that school work seemed improved, both at the time of the initial separation and a year later. A little over a quarter of the mothers saw a negative effect at both time periods, particularly among their sons. For example, both Carol Crossland and Sheryl Stone commented on how their sons were having trouble in school, "acting out" and not paying attention. Sheryl said her son's behavior was improving, however. Carol had begun taking her son to a counselor. On the other hand, only 10% at the early time period and 5% at the later time period said that schoolwork was a *lot* worse.

With regard to their children's relationships, most mothers felt there had been little impact on the children's friendships at either period. In the early period, 20% and, in the later period, 10% mentioned some negative effect (including Carol Crossland, who felt her ex-spouse's several moves at the beginning of the separation, and her own move after a year, had made it hard for her daughter to see her old friends as often as she used to). Fifteen percent said that their children's relationships with friends had improved as a result of the separation ("My daughter doesn't worry about asking to go play with the other kids now," commented Elaine Elkin).

With regard to siblings, the effects seemed more mixed. Almost half the mothers saw no impact on sibling relationships at either time period. However, about 25% felt siblings' relationships had been negatively affected by the separation ("They're always fighting," complained Ms. Nelson, "particularly when they come back from their dad's"), while about an equal proportion felt siblings' relationships had improved ("They're much closer now," observed Carol Crossland. "Maybe because they're together more often, but they really seem to love each other in a nicer way. There's just little things they do together I hadn't seen before—like she'll read to him at bedtime now."). When asked, many children with siblings said they didn't think having siblings had made a difference in helping them get used to the divorce ("No one makes it better," Nancy Nelson replied to the sibling question).

The factors that determine whether a separation will negatively affect relationships with friends or siblings are undoubtedly complicated by the nature of the relationships prior to separation, as well as other factors such as whether the children have to move out of their neighborhood. In any case, it is interesting to note that only about 20% of the children said they talked to friends *or* siblings about the separation, although 80% of the children said they knew other kids whose parents were divorced. Unlike their parents, the children did not seek or find much solace in interpersonal relationships with their siblings or outside the family, though they may have in their relationships with their parents.

Parents were asked to describe any major changes they saw in their children during the postseparation period. Where they felt change had occurred, it was usually seen as positive, consistent with children's self-reports on the standard measures, as well as teacher and parent reports. For example, 39% of the mothers said their children's personality and/or behavior had improved, 19% felt the children's relationship with them had improved, and 13% felt their children's relationship with their father had improved. Nancy Nelson's mother observed that "Nancy's whole attitude is better. I think it helps that I stopped telling her all about my troubles; she doesn't seem so burdened." Elaine Elkin thought that her daughter was feeling more relaxed, because she [her mother] felt more relaxed: "We don't have to rush home, worry about getting there late and her father being mad." Fathers had less to say about perceived changes for their children; however, 25% felt their children's personality had improved and 9% mentioned that fewer resources were available to their children. Christopher Crossland felt that it was good for his children to see that there are "different ways to live. They'll have richer lives knowing that—it's important for kids to see adults being true to themselves."

CHILDREN'S VIEWS OF THEIR PARENTS IN THE POSTSEPARATION PERIOD

Children were asked in both interviews to talk about how they felt their parents were reacting to the separation and divorce. Interestingly, they were perfectly clear that their parents' feelings and reactions were different from their own. For example, though Sally Stone described herself as "sad," she said her parents "aren't sad but they aren't really excited. About the same except they aren't fighting. It's better."

During the initial separation period, a little over half the children described their mothers' reaction as negative. Almost as many (44%) described their mothers' reaction in mostly or totally positive terms. A year later, almost three-quarters described their mothers' reaction in a positive way. Children's descriptions of their fathers' feelings were similar, with 35% describing their fathers as reacting positively at the early period, and 68% at the later period. When asked what they based their answers on, children often said because their parents "told" them. Others inferred their parents' feelings: Nancy Nelson said her mother was happy because "she didn't have to listen to [my] father's yelling and screaming" and that her father "probably feels good because he can go out whenever he wants." Sam Stone said of his father, "I think he feels perfectly fine. He and his girlfriend act like they're married." Of his mother, Sam said, "She just *acts* a lot happier!"

The children who described their mothers' initial reaction as positive were more likely to have had violent fathers, and their mothers were more likely to have initiated the divorce. At the same time, the divorces in these families were less likely to have been mutually planned and more likely to have come about through an impulsive action. This suggests that the mothers in these families may have taken decisive action about a bad situation, perhaps giving them more certainty and confidence, and resulting in their children seeing them as strong and doing well (perhaps as benevolent authorities who could meet their needs as is consistent with the receptive stance). Children who described their mothers' reactions as positive were also more likely to have experienced previous parental separations and were more likely themselves to have had problems in the past, some of which may have been connected to the tension in the marriage.

Children who saw their mothers as reacting primarily negatively to the separation also said the hardest thing for them to get used to was the absence of their father. Their mothers were more likely to have thought about divorce earlier in the marriage and were more likely to be experiencing disapproval from relatives and friends regarding the divorce. In these families, both mothers and children seemed "stuck"—unhappy about their situation and unable to transform it into something more positive. The fact that these mothers were less able to get support from their social network may have rendered them less effective in helping their children cope with their losses.

Children were also asked about how their parents got along together, and they saw some modest improvement in that area as well. We noted above that Sally Stone said her parents "aren't fighting. It's better." Forty-four percent of the children described their parents' interactions as mostly or totally negative at the time of the initial separation, and 36% saw them that way a year later. Although this is not much of a change, it is important to note that 33% of the parents' relationships were described as *totally* negative in the first time period, compared with 18% by the second period.

It is also interesting that the children's perception of their parents' relationship is somewhat more positive than the mothers' own assessment. This may reflect the success of separated parents' efforts to reduce their conflicts in front of the children. Although children as a group were somewhat more positive than mothers over time, within families they tended to see things pretty much the way their parents did. For example, both Carol and Christopher Crossland saw their relationship as strained—Carl Crossland (the 8-year-old) said it was "bad!" Nora Nelson had said her relationship with Ned Nelson was like a "see-saw" depending on what they talked about, and Nancy described it as "sometimes good, sometimes bad." The clarity and consistency of children's accounts of their parents' responses and behaviors (like mothers' reports of their children's) is striking. Both parents and children in separating families were conscious of, and concerned about, each other's adaptation to the new family situation.

CONCLUSIONS

Only a few of the concepts discussed in Chapter 1 (trauma, loss, stigma, risk, life stress, life change, family change, and gender) seemed very pertinent to children's experience of their parents' separation and divorce. Although the experience may have been traumatic in a few cases, mostly it was not. Similarly, most children knew other children whose parents were divorced and did not seem to feel social anxiety or stigma about their parents' separation (though certainly a few did). The children generally showed improved adjustment over time and did not seem to suffer extreme psychological or behavioral disruption, at least in this time frame. The experience did involve loss to a substantial degree, and the concepts of life stress, life change, and family change also apply, though they lack much explanatory force.

There were only a few indications of a gendered response to the separation. For example, boys did seem to "act out" more at school than girls (according to their mothers), and mothers felt that the boys missed their fathers more; in addition, mothers were more likely to report that girls talked about the separation with them. These few differences, though, must be seen against the backdrop of the many emotional and other responses for which there were no gender differences. Overall, children's emotional and behavioral experience of parental separation and divorce were *not* particularly gendered. We suspect that the gender issues arise much less in this domain, and much more in terms of children's beliefs about the implications of their parents' marital and occupational roles for themselves, and in the household practices that dominated the pre- and postseparation households. We will have an opportunity to explore some of these notions in later chapters.

In contrast to the conventional concepts used to think about divorce, which seemed only minimally useful (with the exception of loss), Stewart's account of the receptive stance adopted after major life changes described the children's experience of parental separation quite well. Most children's reports of their early experience (and their parents' reports about them) were dominated by themes of loss and passivity. The themes of autonomy and assertion that were so present in the parents' accounts were not so obvious in the children's, but within 18 months after the separation most children could think of things that were better in the household and perceived both of their parents to be happier. Although it is impossible to ignore the pain the children in these families experienced, it is clear that the process of divorce also freed many of them from some terrible pressures in the preseparation family. Ironically, it also provided them with some "opportunities" that they and their parents recognized: to renegotiate some of their relationships with family members and to observe their parents grappling with and surviving a difficult life crisis. Both the problematic and the beneficial effects of the parental divorce for both the parents and children would no doubt be better understood from a greater distance in time.

Finally, it is important to note that, by comparing children's experiences of parental separation with their parents', we discover that this apparently "shared" family change is in fact profoundly different for the adults and the children involved. Parents have usually spent months or years evaluating the possibility of separation; children almost never have, even in the most violent and unhappy households. Instead, at the moment of separation, when parents must mobilize their efforts to reorganizing their lives and their households, children are coping with sad and surprising news. They are in some very important ways "out of synch" with each other; part of the process of adjustment includes managing these differences in their experience at a time when they very much need each other.

Our task in the remainder of this book is to explore the conditions under which this difficult period in a family's life was relatively more or less difficult for the various members of the family. We know that some of the suffering in this early period is probably inevitable. All family members must recognize what they have lost, and that recognition must bring sadness and distress. Nevertheless, some children, some parents, and some families struggled longer, and with less positive outcomes, than others. It seems to us important to try to identify those things that ease the pain, or result in more benefit in terms of personal growth, as well as those things that merely re-open or deepen the wound.

NOTES

1. As with the parents' accounts in the previous chapter, children's and parents' interviews were coded for particular themes as described in the text. All coding took place with interviews from the 2 years mixed together. Coders were required to attain .85 interrater reliability at the beginning of the coding process, and systematic double coding ensured that all of the coding was completed to that standard of reliability.

2. See Healy, Stewart, and Copeland (1993) for a more complete discussion of the issue of self-blame in children's adjustment to parental separation.

3. These results were all significant beyond the $p < .05$ level.

PART TWO

HOW INDIVIDUAL FAMILY MEMBERS ADAPT TO PARENTAL SEPARATION

In this section we examine the factors that made the process of adjustment to parental separation easier or harder. Our focus in these two chapters is on parents and children as individuals.

In Chapter 5, we examine parents' adjustment after the separation. We find that there are two distinct phases. In the early period, the factors that help are those that help parents address the concrete tasks involved with establishing and maintaining the new household. In the later period, the factors that help are those that help parents find satisfying interpersonal relationships and develop themselves.

In Chapter 6, we examine children's adjustment after the separation. One of the most important things we find is that very few factors are uniformly helpful or harmful to children's adjustment. Parental conflict was generally hard on children, and social understanding skills were helpful, particularly in the early period. But most other findings depended very much on which group of children we were considering. For example, both mothers' employment and postseparation school and household changes had very different effects for children of different ages or sexes.

The findings for individual parents and children underscore the ways in which all family members are embedded in relationships inside the family and outside it. This section therefore paves the way for our consideration of family dyads in Part III.

CHAPTER 5

Parents Adjusting after the Separation
WHAT HELPED?

We have seen that in the course of parental separation both parents and children make fairly dramatic emotional adjustments. There is evidence that for both distress decreases over time, and that a process of emotional adaptation is marked by an initial focus on competence for the parents, and passive receptivity for the children. One scholar has argued that in negotiating any major life transition people face two different kinds of tasks: solving concrete or practical problems, and addressing more personal psychological needs (Golan, 1983). As we saw in Chapter 3, the parents in our study did focus on the specific tasks involved in setting up and maintaining the postseparation households during the immediate period following the separation. Later, they showed more interest in other issues, including their personal growth and establishing new emotional and relational ties.

If these were the critical tasks facing parents in the process of separation and divorce, any factors in their lives that helped them work on these tasks should have facilitated their adjustment to this life transition. We found, particularly in the case of our mothers, that circumstances that supported concrete problem solving or that allowed the mothers to feel competent to handle their lives did seem to help early on. While the benefit of some of these factors persisted over the year after separation, other factors, specifically related to the mothers' interpersonal relationships with friends and relatives, as well as their ex-spouses, were especially important as mothers began to ad-

This chapter was drafted by Janet E. Malley.

dress their more personal and relational needs. The results in this chapter support the impression we gained in Chapter 3 that in the early phase parents need support in immediate, day-to-day demands of establishing a household and family routine, whereas later they need support for more personal and psychological concerns. One mother in our study was clearly quite aware of this process. She responded to our question about her future plans in the first interview, "I don't have any long-term goals right now. Right now my only goals are getting this family raised. . . . After that, then I'll think about more future for myself."

We have much richer and more complete data on many aspects of the households with children than those without them (we have several reporters on the households with children). Because mothers were the custodial parents in so many of the postseparation households with children, we have much more evidence about the factors that helped mothers adjust in the postseparation period. We included all custodial mothers who participated in either interview session; fathers who participated both years were included, regardless of whether they were living with or apart from their children. Because the sample of fathers is small and reflects quite varied household compositions, we view our findings about their postseparation adjustment as quite provisional. We will discuss them separately at the end of the chapter.

WHAT HELPED MOTHERS ADJUST?

We tried to identify aspects of the women's lives and personalities that might, separately or in combination, affect their ability to address the tasks they faced. We looked for factors relevant to their ability to establish and maintain their new postseparation household in the early transition period and, later, those factors related to their more personal concerns about growth and interpersonal relationships. These factors are listed in Table 5.1.

In terms of resources for meeting day-to-day demands, we thought having *paid employment* would be especially beneficial to women in the early period, not only for the regular income it provided to support their family and household needs, but also for its potential to afford the women a feeling of competence and knowledge that they could handle the instrumental tasks they were facing at home. This sense of competence might be especially likely for women employed in relatively *high-status occupations*. In contrast, there were also barriers to support for day-to-day demands. For example, employed mothers who felt *pulled between work and family demands*, as well as those mothers who experienced a *worsening financial situation postseparation*, might be realistically apprehensive about their ability to manage and maintain their new single-parent household.

We also considered the mothers' social networks as a source of both

TABLE 5.1. Factors Associated with Mothers' Adjustment

Factors affecting support for mothers' day-to-day demands

Resources for meeting demands
- Preseparation paid employment
  Preschool children in family
  Adolescent children in family
- Higher job status (socioeconomic status)
  High interparent conflict
  High legal conflict
- Practical help
  Mother employed full-time
  High legal conflict

Obstacles to meeting demands
- Worsened financial situation
  Preschool children in family
- Work–family conflict
  Preschool children in family
  Divorce not settled by Time 2

Factors affecting support for mothers' psychological growth

Resources for growth
- Emotional support
  Mother not employed full-time
- Affiliation motivation
- Dating

Obstacles to growth
- Conflict with ex-spouse
- Power motivation

Note. Italics denote subgroups showing significant effects for this factor.

practical help (support for day-to-day demands) for more immediate household management and *emotional support* (support for psychological growth) as mothers moved on to address their more general psychosocial needs. Friends and family members were often available to the mothers, especially in the early transition period, for both financial and task assistance (e.g., babysitting, car maintenance, etc.), directly benefiting the mothers' early efforts to establish and manage their new households. These interpersonal relationships could also be beneficial to the mothers later on as a source of emotional support for the mothers. In contrast, prolonged *negative interactions with their ex-husbands* could interfere with these efforts toward personal growth and interpersonal connectedness, and impede prospects for their longer-term adjustment.

Finally, we thought characteristics within the mothers themselves might also play a role in their ability to address these two important tasks associated with major life transitions. Some personality characteristics might be either resources for coping with these new demands or liabilities making coping more difficult. Specifically, we suspected that those women who were high in an underlying *need for power* might be particularly frustrated, because divorce might threaten their prestige and influence, which are highly valued commodities for people with a high power motive. In contrast, women expressing a high *need for affiliation,* usually associated with feelings of loneliness and a desire for close friendly relations, might have more difficulty addressing their need for warm, companionate relations in the context of divorce.

We identified, then, two sets of factors in these women's lives that we thought should have some impact on their ability to adjust to their separation and divorce: factors that facilitated or impeded their ability to tackle the concrete, day-to-day demands they faced in the early postseparation period; and factors that aided or detracted from their effort to address their personal psychological needs. Whereas more demographic characteristics of the family (e.g., number, ages, and gender of the children) are often thought to be important, we found that such family differences had little relevance to mothers' divorce adjustment.

The factors we identified as important in this postseparation period are reported for the entire mother sample as well as for some subgroups of mothers that showed specific relationships of these factors to mothers' adjustment. We will begin by focusing on the adjustment of all mothers living with their children, the largest group for whom we have the most complete data; where relevant, we will also explore some subgroups of women with particular problems or resources that seemed to directly affect their ability to address the tasks associated with this transition period. Finally, we will turn to a discussion of the fathers' postseparation adjustment.

We will examine the relationships of these variables to adjustment within each time for the two data collection periods. In addition, we will explore relations between Time 1 factors and Time 2 adjustment. Over-time analyses of this sort are helpful in two ways. They may help identify factors that are irrelevant to short-term adjustment but have longer-term benefits (or costs). Thus, emotional support may help keep a person aware of how painful the divorce is in the short term; over the longer term, though, having experienced those painful feelings fully may permit a process of "working through" that enhances eventual adjustment. Second, some factors that are associated with adjustment within time may actually reflect relationships "caused" by adjustment; for example, if practical help is related to better adjustment, this could be because having help makes mothers feel better, or it could be because mothers who are better adjusted are more effective at getting practical help. When we examine over-time correlations, we can sometimes clarify our understanding of the relationships. If being helped at Time 1 is also connected with better adjustment at Time 2, we can be more confident that it is the help that is producing better adjustment. Generally, we did not have as much information from the fathers; thus, we were not able to examine as many characteristics of their lives as we did with the mothers.[1]

Support for Day-to-Day Demands in the Early Postseparation Period and Mothers' Adjustment

Table 5.2 summarizes the statistically significant relationships between factors affecting the mothers' ability to address the new, day-to-day demands of running a single-parent household at Time 1 and their immediate (Time 1) and longer-term (Time 2) adjustment. Overall, it is clear that aspects of mothers' employment and job-based socioeconomic status were related to their psychological well-being at Time 1 and their physical health over time. Practical help was associated with better psychological and physical health at Time 1 and continued better physical health over time, while perceived improvement in the financial situation provided only short-term psychological benefit for some women.

TABLE 5.2. Correlations between Support for Day-to-Day Demands at Time 1 and Mothers' Adjustment

	Time 1		Time 2	
	Psychological adjustment	Physical illness	Psychological adjustment	Physical illness
Preseparation paid employment	+			−
Preschool children in family	+	−		−
Adolescent children in family	+			
Higher job status (socioeconomic status)	+			−
High interparent conflict	+		+	−
Worsened financial situation				
Preschool children in family	−			
Practical help	+	−		−
Mother employed full-time	+	−		
High legal conflict	+	−		

Note. Italics denote subgroups showing significant effects for this factor. + indicates that the characteristic is assessed with a higher score on either adjustment (a positive indicator) or illness (a negative indicator); − indicates that the characteristic is assessed with a lower score on either adjustment (a negative indicator) or illness (a positive indicator).

Mothers' Preseparation Employment

For the sample of mothers as a whole, having paid employment[2] prior to the separation was related to good adjustment at Time 1. Paid employment may help distract a woman from problems in her family life, offer her financial and psychological rewards, and provide her with a network of relationships. Continuous paid employment also played a role in predicting good physical health for the mothers at Time 2, suggesting that the positive aspects of working had long-term effects as well during this stressful period. Having no paid employment was clearly problematic for divorcing mothers. However, having to take on employment as a *new* role during an already stressful period apparently exacerbated the psychological and physical distress the mothers were already experiencing. A new job for a woman who has been out of the labor force is unlikely to provide either the financial or the psychological rewards associated with employment in a position for which she is experienced and feels well qualified.

Moreover, the effects of paid employment in the preseparation period varied, depending on the complexity of the age structure of the household. For example, already having paid employment at the time of separation played a much stronger role in predicting good psychological (Time 1) and physical health (Time 2) among mothers whose families included preschool children and better psychological health (Time 1) for those whose families included adolescents than among mothers who only had children between 6 and 12 years old. Families with children of very different ages (school-age and either much younger or much older) may be both draining to manage full-time, and particularly complicated to schedule. Mothers who had already worked out routines for handling their own work schedules no doubt had an advantage over women who had not developed such routines because they either were not employed or had only recently become employed. In addition, the children who already had experience with their mothers' employment were not faced with this additional change in their lives as compared to children whose mothers took on paid employment in this early postseparation period.

Mothers of adolescent children who had been at home full-time before the separation also may have been uncomfortable leaving them alone for the first time after the separation. One nonemployed mother of three children expressed to us her worry about what would happen if she did get a job and her oldest, teenage daughter was left in charge at home: "If she were home . . . it would just be mass murder. They don't get along whatsoever."

In addition, mothers of very young children who only began paid employment in response to the divorce may have felt some guilt associated with such a move, particularly if the reason they were not gainfully employed prior to their separation was so they could be home for their young children. A mother of three young children who was having a particularly difficult time during this early separation period did find herself in a quandary about working, because she needed the money, but also felt she needed to be home for her children:

> "Financially it's just like I'm in poverty and a few times through the past year I've been like, in a panic and going to get a job, and it was Michelle's counselor who said to me that I [should] not get a job because right now my priorities are my kids. . . . So I've had a difficult time, but now it's, like, I have to get a job. And I'm making it so it's on weekends and their father will take care of them. . . . So I'm trying to do it so that I don't interfere with them, their home life."

In contrast, another mother of similarly young children who had an established career prior to her separation vividly described how important her job was to her, particularly during this difficult time in her life:

> "Initially, it was the only thing I had to hang on to. It was the only area that I felt competent. I felt like I was a failure as a mother, a failure as a wife, a woman. And it was the only area where I knew I could go every day and people would say, 'You're doing a good job.'"

Moreover, by this time she found her kids had "adjusted pretty well to the work."

Job Status (Socioeconomic Status)

Paid employment in higher-status jobs involving more prestige, income, and responsibilities was also associated with well-being at Time 1.[3] Undoubtedly the greater financial resources accompanying higher-status jobs helped relieve some of the monetary strain normally associated with divorce, making the adjustment process less stressful for these women. In addition, a higher-status job may more often provide women with a sense of achievement and competence that they can then bring into the family arena. As one mother told us:

> "I wanted to work for the self-satisfaction. I still want to work for the self-satisfaction. The money's very nice, but I enjoy work. I get something out of it. . . . I feel good about me when I'm working. I mean I could sit home very nicely all day long and collect welfare or make his

support go up 10 times higher than he [pays] right now and just sit around and do what I want to do for myself, but I do get a lot out of working."

We can be fairly confident that it is higher status that affects well-being rather than the reverse, because being employed in a job with higher socioeconomic status at Time 1 continued to benefit women 1 year later, in terms of their better physical health.

In the early postseparation period, women in higher-status jobs who experienced high levels of conflict with their ex-husbands were also better adjusted than women in lower-status jobs facing these same circumstances. The women in higher-status jobs may have felt more financially and personally independent, and they may have had more confidence in their ability to handle the divorce process and to pay the legal expenses associated with a fair settlement.

Perceived Change in Financial Situation

We have already noted that mothers in higher-status (and better paying) jobs were better off psychologically than mothers in lower-status jobs. We also directly assessed mothers' perceptions of the postseparation change in their financial situation on a 3-point scale: things got better, things stayed the same, things got worse (based on mothers' responses to a direct question asked in the interview, "Would you say your financial situation changed after the separation?"). Perception of postseparation changes in women's financial situation was not associated with their divorce adjustment at either Time 1 or Time 2. This is a little surprising, especially because for most of the women in our sample (as in other studies; see Kurz, 1995, and Peterson, 1989) the level of financial resources declined with marital separation. We were, however, struck by the number of women who did not express distress over this change, despite recognizing it. Many women were, in fact, pleased with their new financial situation, primarily because, although they had less money available to support the family, it was money over which they had direct control. One mother told us:

> "Well, there's less money coming into our house because of his money, but I think the bills are being better paid. I'm finding it very, very different, but I like being in charge of paying the bills."

However, we did find that perceiving their financial situation as worse than before was strongly associated with poorer psychological adjustment at Time 1 for women with young children. These mothers may have been particularly concerned about how they could provide financially for their families' needs and still be available to care for their young children.

Practical Help

If a major component of parents' adjustment involved being able to address the immediate, practical demands of family life, then concrete help parents received from those outside the family should also make a difference. In describing their typical weekdays and weekends mothers often mentioned the help with child care and other tasks related to household and family responsibilities (such as meals, errands, yard work, car care, etc.) they received from friends and extended family members. The interviews were scored for mothers mentioning that they received such help from friends and relatives.[4]

As we expected, mothers' reports of practical help from their social network were associated with both psychological and physical well-being in the early period; the mothers definitely benefited when they had outside help managing their households, a job they once shared with their husbands. Such assistance was particularly valuable to women who were working full-time and those who were experiencing high levels of legal conflict with their ex-husbands. These subgroups represent women whose divorce experiences may have been especially complicated and/or stressful and the tasks associated with early divorce adjustment even more demanding. Although the availability of outside help in the early period was apparently useful in alleviating some of the pressures the women experienced early in the divorce process, this early help did not provide as much long-term benefit, although it continued to be associated with better health at Time 2.

To summarize, factors in the early postseparation period that enabled women to deal effectively with the practicalities of their households were associated with better functioning at Time 1. Support that actually provided the mothers in our study with material help facilitated their early psychological and physical adjustment. Similarly, experiences that supported their feelings of competence as well as their ability to provide financially for their families, such as stable employment (particularly in high-status, high-paying jobs) were also associated with well-being in this early period of study.

Support for Day-to-Day Demands and Mothers' Adjustment in the Later Postseparation Period

By 18 months postseparation very few indicators of material support were related to mothers' divorce adjustment. Perhaps the mothers had had sufficient time to establish a single-parent household so that day-to-day family operations were less directly tied to their feelings of well-being. However, in instances where many of the details of family organization were still being worked out at Time 2, particularly when mothers were experiencing conflict between household and employment needs or were still in conflict with their ex-spouses about the divorce settlement, support for day-to-day responsibilities still had an impact on mothers' adjustment. Table 5.3 summarizes relationships between Time 2 support for day-to-day demands and mothers' adjustment.

Mothers' Employment

Paid employment by Time 2 was not associated with well-being for our mothers (perhaps because nearly 90% of the women were employed either full- or part-time by then); however, the advantage of higher-status employment for working mothers persisted at Time 2 for the mothers who were experiencing higher levels of legal conflict with their ex-husbands. These women were physically healthier than women experiencing similar conflict but employed in lower-status jobs.

Mothers' Experience of Work–Family Conflict

Although paid employment at Time 2 was not directly related to mothers' adjustment, it was problematic for mothers who felt particularly conflicted

TABLE 5.3. Correlations between Support for Day-to-Day Demands and Mothers' Adjustment within Time 2

	Time 2	
	Psychological adjustment	Physical illness
Paid employment		
Higher job status (socioeconomic status)		
High legal conflict		–
Worsened financial situation		
Work–family conflict	–	
Preschool children in family	–	
Divorce not settled by Time 2	–	
Practical help		

Note. Italics and + and – signs as in Table 5.2.

about the competing demands of work and children. Work–family conflict was coded as present or absent according to mothers' responses to a direct interview question ("Often parents who are working experience conflict between their work responsibilities and parenting responsibilities. Does this happen for you?"). This question was only asked at Time 2 when we gathered more detailed information about the mothers' work experiences.

Work–family conflict was particularly problematic if the mothers had young children or if the terms of the divorce had not yet been settled by Time 2. Both of these situations can prolong and/or intensify the uncertainty typical of the postseparation period, making it more difficult for these mothers to address the day-to-day demands they faced and move on to attending to their own intrapsychic needs.

Support for Psychological and Relationship Growth

Once mothers had established a relatively smoothly functioning set of household arrangements after the separation, we expected them to focus on their personal needs for psychological growth and warm, personal relationships. In this period support for, and obstacles to, their adjustment should come from different sources. We expected emotional support from friends and relatives, dating relationships, and affiliation motivation to support adjustment, and conflict with the ex-spouses and power motivation to interfere with it. Table 5.4 summarizes the relationships between Time 1 support for psychological and relationship growth and mothers' adjustment within time (Time 1) and over time (Time 2); Table 5.5 reports on these relationships within Time 2.

TABLE 5.4. Correlations between Time 1 Support for Psychological and Relationship Growth and Mothers' Adjustment, Time 1 and Time 2

Time 1	Time 1		Time 2	
	Psychological adjustment	Physical illness	Psychological adjustment	Physical illness
Emotional support			+	
Mother not employed full-time			+	−
Affiliation motivation				
Conflict with ex-spouse				+
Power motivation			−	+

Note. Italics and + and − signs as in Table 5.2.

TABLE 5.5. Correlations between Time 2 Support for Psychological and Relationship Growth and Mothers' Adjustment, Time 2

	Time 2	
	Psychological adjustment	Physical illness
Emotional support		
Affiliation motivation		
Dating	+	−
Conflict with ex-spouse		
Power motivation	−	+

Note. + and − signs as in Table 5.2.

Emotional Support

Using a questionnaire we labeled "talking with others," we asked parents to indicate how much (on a 3-point scale: 1 = not at all; 2 = only generally in the last 6 months; 3 = in great detail in the last 6 months) they had discussed eight general issues or concerns (such as things that made them furious or worried, financial difficulties, how they felt about the divorce, concerns about their children, and hopes for the future) with family members, friends, or professionals such as counselors or social workers. Emotional support scores summed the amount each woman had recently talked about all of these topics with friends and relatives in her network.

Emotional support from friends and relatives (measured by self-report of time spent talking with friends or relatives about personal concerns) during the early postseparation period was *not* related to their early divorce adjustment. However, by Time 2, it was associated with better psychological adjustment for the total sample of mothers; this over-time finding helps confirm our view that these interpersonal relationships were of some benefit to the mothers, particularly later in this transition period when they were able to focus on their more psychological concerns. One mother explained that

> "talking to people is an outlet. The guy I share an office with was invaluable in the past year. He was one of the first people to know there were problems and that I was probably going to get a divorce. And he was really the only one who knew for a long time, but just having someone to be able to talk to about it . . . he's been a very good friend in that respect."

The relationship between emotional support and the mothers' psychological well-being was not present within Time 2, suggesting that having such support early on is critical to the mothers, even though the benefit is not immediately evident. These interpersonal relationships were particularly valuable for women who were not employed full-time and thus perhaps had fewer structured opportunities to interact with others; they demonstrated both better psychological and better physical health by Time 2 than similar mothers without such support.

Dating

We did not assess dating behavior in the early postseparation period; however, women who were dating by Time 2 were higher in psychological and physical well-being than women who were not in a dating relationship. One mother, who was not dating, talked of how she wished she had such a relationship, "I miss just having companionship. . . . Now I just feel as though, you know, sometimes I wish I had somebody there to talk to, you know?" Another mother described her live-in boyfriend as her "partner. He is my friend. He's my lover. He's my partner. I want that to continue. . . . I want to be more his friend and to be a part of him and him a part of me."

Affiliation Motivation

Surprisingly, affiliation motivation—or the desire for warm, companionate relations with others[5]—was unrelated to the mothers' divorce adjustment at both times. In previous research, affiliation motivation has been found to be associated with two kinds of interpersonal patterns: high levels of sociability and interpersonal involvement and a tendency toward loneliness and unpopularity (see Koestner & McClelland, 1992, for a summary of the literature). Although the desire for close, friendly relations might be viewed as threatened by the situation of divorce, perhaps mothers with custody of their children had sufficient access to such relations, both with their children and through the network of friends and family they retained.

Conflict with Ex-Spouses

From both the parents' and children's interviews we were able to assess the level of conflict between the parents as viewed by each family member interviewed. Specifically, parents were asked, "What would you say is the state of your relationship with your spouse now?" Similarly, children in the family were asked, "Now that your parents are not living together anymore, how do they get along when they talk to each other?" These individual answers were coded along a 5-point scale from 1 = no overt conflict/tension to 5 = constant overt conflict/tension. One parent, whose response was coded for constant conflict/tension, described her relationship with her husband as

> "not very good. The divorce doesn't work, it's the pits. Hostility, resentment. We have very little interaction, if any. It goes nowhere. There's either no interaction or there is haggling. It is totally frustrating."

Characteristic of the midpoint of the scale (episodic or sporadic conflict) was another parental response to this question: "Basically pretty good. On all the big stuff and the hard stuff there have been really no problems. Picky little details, I thought he was a pain in the neck." And at the other extreme of the conflict scale (no overt tension or conflict) is this parent's answer: "There are occasions when common business has to be attended to, and it's done on a very friendly basis."

Responses for each interviewed family member were scored according to the same 5-point scale.[6] These scores were then averaged to create a parental conflict score, based on multiple reporters. Like emotional support, conflict with their ex-spouses in the early postseparation period was not related to mothers' divorce adjustment. Parents probably expect a significant level of conflict when they begin the divorce process, so its presence at that time may not interfere with their adjustment.

However, early conflict *was* associated with poorer physical health by Time 2. These results suggest that the stress associated with such conflict may accumulate, eventually wearing the mothers down; over time mothers who experienced higher levels of early conflict with their ex-spouses apparently reacted to this stress with physical health problems.

Power Motivation

Power motivation is a social motive relevant to many of the issues divorcing parents face. Generally, "power motivation" is defined as an underlying wish or desire to have an impact on others; it is often not at all conscious, and it may be expressed in behavior designed to gain attention or prestige, as well as in efforts to influence, persuade, or lead others (see Winter, 1973, 1992). Men and women differ in the consequences of the power motive for intimate relationships (Stewart & Rubin, 1974; Winter, 1988, 1992). Previous research has shown that men high in power motivation tend to have difficulties in relationships, are more likely to get divorced, and approach women with an eye to conquest rather than intimacy. In contrast, women high in power motivation are not especially prone to relationship difficulties; in fact, they may view relationships as vehicles for prestige. As a result, they may be especially unhappy with the situation of divorce, in which their social value or prestige is reduced. (See Stewart & Chester, 1982, and Winter, 1988, 1992, for accounts of the correlates of power motivation in men and women.)

Not surprisingly, then, we found that mothers' Time 1 power motivation[7] was associated with poorer physical and psychological well-being by Time 2. Given the importance power-motivated individuals attach to prestige and status, the loss of a social role society has endowed with particular status for women may have been particularly stressful for these women. One such mother said to us:

> "I wouldn't go into McDonald's and have a cup of coffee by myself 'cause they might say, 'Oh, she's all alone,' right? That's a little thing that's been hard to get used to. Although [before the separation] I went many places alone with the children, I knew my husband was at home so I never felt alone. When I go places with the children now and I know there's no husband home, it is, 'Gee, I don't have anybody at home. I look unmarried, right?'"

This relationship between power motivation and adjustment in the mothers suggests that, over time, the loss of the marital relationship was especially damaging for power-motivated women. For example, a mother in our study who characterized herself as an "old-fashioned," full-time mother felt threatened by the time her children spent with their dad:

> "I get aggravated . . . when the kids get on the phone with their father. They tie up my phone for over an hour at a time, and they talk to him most every night. . . . And I find that I resent them being on the phone with him. . . . I feel they see him quite a bit. They don't call me when they're gone for the weekend. . . . I still am very angry with him. I feel that he's the biggest phony that ever walked down the pike. That all of a sudden, once he moved out, he took interest in his children which he didn't do before. And I can't help but [think] it's a phony interest."

Whereas many of the mothers in our study were pleased with, and usually encouraged, their ex-husbands' contact with their children, this mother resented the time her children spent with their father, even if much of that time was limited to phone conversations. This resentment appears to stem, in part, from the loss of power and control over the remaining family members in her household. Not only is this power-motivated mother experiencing the loss of power she had in her marital relationship, but the level of control she has in her relationship with her children also feels tenuous.

Power motivation at Time 2 was also associated with poor psychological well-being for the mothers, as well as poorer physical health. For this group of women, divorce seems to pose a substantial adaptive challenge, one they have not met well, at least within the time frame of this study.

WHAT HELPED FATHERS ADJUST?

As noted before, the fathers in our sample differed in the degree to which they were managing households with children or not. However, the total sample was too small to explore these two groups of fathers separately. Because we suspect that the issues raised for adjustment under these two conditions may be very different, we provide analyses of the factors that helped or hindered fathers' adjustment in our sample with caution. In addition, because noncustodial parents were not asked to provide as much information as custodial parents, we have fewer measures of potentially important factors for the fathers than we did for the mothers. Table 5.6 summarizes the relationships between variables and fathers' adjustment at both times.

Support for Day-to-Day Demands

Although many of the instrumental support factors explored with the mother sample could not be examined in the father sample, job status could be. In contrast with the mothers, job status was marginally related to fathers' *poorer* psychological well-being by Time 2. Given the higher social status of men, in general, than women, perhaps it is not surprising that having a high-status job did not confer psychological benefits on men in the way it did on women in the divorcing process. In fact, for men in higher-income (and higher-sta-

TABLE 5.6. Correlations between Support Variables and Adjustment for Fathers

	Time 1		Time 2	
Time 1	Psychological adjustment	Physical illness	Psychological adjustment	Physical illness
Job status Time 1			(−)	
Emotional support Time 1		+		+
Emotional support Time 2				(+)
Dating Time 2			(+)	
Affiliation motivation Time 1	−			
Affiliation motivation Time 2			(−)	

Note. + and − signs as in Table 5.2. ( ) indicates relationships that are not statistically significant but suggest a trend.

tus) occupations, in contrast to those in occupations with lesser status and income, losing a wife may have implied losses of career resources (including, e.g., help with social events and occasions), successful self-image, and prestige that were important in sustaining men in these positions. These lost resources were apparently not trivial, as the negative relationship between employment status and psychological well-being persisted over time.

Support for Psychological and Relationship Growth

Whereas emotional support (or talking a lot to other people) was unrelated to mothers' early divorce adjustment it was associated with the fathers' *poorer* physical health at Time 1. It appears that for fathers, talking to others did *not* provide them with emotional support needed for their adjustment. Instead, perhaps distressed fathers felt more of a need to talk to others (in fact, fathers experiencing higher levels of conflict with their ex-spouses at Time 1 were more likely to be talking to other adults), but did not find other people's responses supportive or helpful. It is unclear whether this resulted from fathers' lesser ability to elicit sympathy and support, or from their networks' inclination to be less supportive or more critical of divorcing men than women. Perhaps men experience the need to discuss personal issues such as divorce as so embarrassing and uncomfortable that the discomfort offsets the emotional support.

Emotional support continued to be associated with fathers' poorer health both over time and at Time 2. Those fathers experiencing stress well into the divorce process continued to talk with others about their problems, but they were unsuccessful in gaining relief or comfort from these interactions. However, like the mothers, fathers who were in dating relationships by Time 2 (fully 84%) demonstrated marginally better psychological adjustment than those who were not.

Unlike the mothers, power motivation was not relevant to the fathers' divorce adjustment. As mentioned earlier, power-motivated men tend to view women as potential "conquests," are likely to have difficulties in relationships, and are often divorced. Moreover, for men the role of divorcé causes less stigma than it does for women. For these reasons, power-motivated men, unlike power-motivated women, may be able to view divorce as providing them with an opportunity to acquire a new relationship with a woman that might offer more prestige than the last one.

As we expected, fathers who were high in affiliation motivation at Time 1 *were* significantly lower on adjustment (unlike mothers with this personality characteristic). For men high in affiliation motivation (like women high in power motivation), divorce may provide an exceptionally frustrating and painful experience, because of its connection with loneliness and isolation.

One father, in recounting to us how he felt when his wife told him she wanted a divorce, said:

> "When she said, 'I'm going to leave you now,' I said, 'I'm afraid I'll never be able to find another woman,' and, gee, it's true. And so, I see the loneliness aspect of it as worse for me. . . . The lack of female companionship is really the hardest thing for me to bear. . . . I do know that I don't want to grow old alone. I just, I dread that very much."

Clearly divorce was very distressing for men like this father. Moreover, marriage may have provided these men not only with an important intimate relationship, but also a network of friendly, social relations. The loss of a marriage partner, then, threatened not only the loss of intimacy and companionship in that relationship, but a whole set of social relations.

Affiliation motivation at Time 2 was also associated with poorer psychological adjustment, although by this time the relationship was only a trend (not statistically significant). The fathers were still feeling some loss of interpersonal relationships that their families had previously provided for them. A year and a half after he moved out one father told us:

> "Some nights I come home and I'm very lonely. And I'll call up the house and I'll say hi to my daughter, and she'll say, 'Dad, I'm busy, I'm watching television. Call me back.' And I feel like saying, 'Who the hell cares about television?' "

COMPARING THE PATTERN FOR
FATHERS AND MOTHERS

Although we view our findings cautiously, the fathers' experience in this early period presented a rather different picture than that of the mothers. Interpersonal relationships were of more importance to the fathers than the mothers early in the divorce process. Distressed fathers seem to have sought support by talking with others about their emotional concerns, but they did not find comfort or a sense of well-being by doing so. In addition, fathers who scored high on affiliation motivation were especially miserable during the early period.

Some factors found to be important to the fathers' adjustment at Time 1 were also relevant at Time 2; however, new factors were also significant. Emotional support and affiliation motivation continued to be negatively associated with fathers' adjustment 18 months after parental separation, suggesting that interpersonal relations continued to be weakly associated with fathers' poorer well-being. Fathers who were most stressed in this period pursued conversation with other adults, but those conversations were still not effective in helping the men to feel better. However, dating relationships at Time 2 did benefit these men psychologically.

CONCLUSIONS

The factors associated with adjustment in the early and later period confirm the structure of mothers' divorce adjustment (or perhaps the divorce adjustment of custodial parents) suggested by the parents' own stories in Chapter 3. In the early postseparation period custodial mothers must focus on the immediate demands associated with a change in household make-up and routine. These demands can range from sorting out who will get what furniture to finding a new place to live, enrolling children in school in a new community, starting or changing jobs, or changing the number of hours of employment. These are such demanding and time-consuming tasks that the women may have needed to direct virtually all of their attention and effort to their completion, leaving very little energy for other aspects of their lives. Aspects of women's lives that supported these efforts, whether through receiving direct help from others, encouraging women's feelings of competence, or providing financial security eased their divorce adjustment in this early period. However, we also found that the personality characteristic of power motivation interfered with their early divorce adjustment. Perhaps for power-motivated women the loss of status and prestige associated with the traditional marital household is a liability they cannot easily overcome. The focus for them is on the loss of power they have suffered, rather than the demands to restructure and reorganize their families.

Over time, as some of the immediate problems were resolved and the family began to function in its new form, most mothers were able to reduce the energy directed toward these practical issues and redirect it into areas of more social or emotional concern for them, facing the other critical set of tasks in negotiating major life transitions. Thus, further into the transition process, how others outside the immediate family responded to them became increasingly important. We found that over time mothers benefited from the emotional support provided by friends and relatives as well as in dating relationships. However, factors that prevented mothers from resolving immediate day-to-day family concerns, such as feeling conflicted about competing work and family responsibilities, and persisting open conflict with their ex-spouses, interfered with their longer-term adjustment.

The fathers in our study presented us with much less specific information about what factors facilitated or impeded the process of divorce adjustment for them. This lack of clarity may have as much to do with the nature of our study as with the difficulties involved in understanding what may be perceived by men as a particularly sensitive and private process for them. The group of fathers we studied was a smaller and more limited sample than our sample of mothers. Fewer of the men than the women we contacted agreed to participate in our study. Although we found no demographic differences between men who agreed to be in the study and those who refused, we suspect that our participating fathers may have been particularly lonely and eager to have the opportunity to talk with someone. Fewer of these fathers, for example, were dating by Time 2 than the ex-husbands of the women we interviewed (at least by their ex-wives' accounts). Moreover, the fathers in our study who were more distressed also tended to seek out more adult companionship. In addition, even though the sample of fathers was smaller than the mothers, the fathers' situations tended to be more variable. In particular, whereas most of the women in our study had physical custody of their children, the fathers represented far more diversity in custody arrangements. With such variability in divorce situations it may be difficult to discover common factors related generally to fathers' adjustment.

Moreover, many of the contextual factors of interest to us in trying to understand the process of divorce adjustment were not specifically pursued with the fathers in mind. For example, as many of our interview questions focused on the daily experience and family routine of the mother-custody household, similar questions directed at noncustodial fathers were not very revealing of their lives. In contrast, we probed very little into experiences at work, which for many men may have represented a far more important realm. (This domain was clearly very important for women, too, but in ways—conflict between work and family, job status, and benefits of paid employment—that were apparently not so relevant for men.)

We did learn, however, that the loss of the marital relationship was especially problematic for fathers who were high in affiliation motivation. While loss of status and prestige was an important factor for some women, it was the loss of an important intimate relationship that was negatively associated with adjustment for some of the fathers. Moreover, we found a strong relationship between poor adjustment in the fathers and pursuing conversations with friends. In the situation of divorce, distressed fathers may be very concerned about developing a social network outside the family to provide the emotional support previously received within the family. Our evidence suggests, though, that at least in the beginning they are not very successful in using that network to their own advantage.

Gender seemed to play a role in shaping both men's and women's adjustment to divorce. Ultimately it appears that for women issues of power were particularly deeply implicated in the adjustment process, whereas for men it was issues of relationships. For example, aspects of paid employment were more important for women, probably partly because it is less sex-role normative for them, and partly because for women—but perhaps not for men—employment is empowering. In fact, although we can't be sure it was a response to the divorce situation, the fact that men in high-status jobs were actually *worse* off psychologically suggests that gendered aspects of employment increase men's vulnerability under some conditions. Similarly, power motivation was associated with more strain for women.

There were large differences in the impact of relationships on women's and men's adjustment. For women, practical help from others was helpful at Time 1, emotional support and dating at Time 2. In addition, conflict with their ex-spouses was problematic. In short, positive relationships had positive effects and negative relationships had negative ones. For men, in contrast, while dating was beneficial, overall the domain of relationships seemed particularly troubled, and not especially helpful.

At the same time, certain aspects of the results do suggest an overall pattern characteristic of both mothers and fathers. In Chapter 3 we found that the early period of separation and divorce for parents was characterized by a strong focus on autonomy and competence, with a secondary preoccupation with loss. In the later period, parents seemed to be in the beginning stages of establishing stable, satisfying relationships and lives for themselves. In parallel fashion, the factors that supported adjustment (at least for mothers) in the early period turned out to be those things that should have helped them to manage the tasks of creating new and effective households and routines for themselves and their children. These factors waned in importance during the later period; instead, the factors that supported adjustment in the later period (for both men and women) were those things likely to have helped them to become more responsive and attentive partners in relationships. Similarly, the things that jeopardized parents' adjustment were factors that interfered with one or the other of these outcomes.

We have seen in Chapters 3 and 4 that children and parents had very different experiences of the process of parental separation and divorce. In the next chapter we will be able to compare the factors that promoted or jeopardized children's adjustment with those that helped and hurt that of their parents.

NOTES

1. Results from these statistical analyses are found in the Appendix. Appendix Table 5.1 presents correlations for the mother sample for Time 1 and over time; Appendix Table 5.2 presents results of mother-data analyses for Time 2. Appendix Table 5.3 presents results of all father-data analyses.

2. Mothers' employment status was coded on a 3-point scale: no paid employment (working less than 5 hours per week); part-time employment (working 5–29 hours per week); full-time employment (30 or more hours per week).

3. Job status was coded according to Hollingshead and Redlich's (1958) code for occupational prestige, from 1 = unskilled workers to 7 = major professionals (e.g., doctors, lawyers, university professors).

4. All coding took place with interviews from the 2 years mixed together. Coders were required to attain .85 interrater reliability at the beginning of the coding process, and systematic double coding ensured that all of the coding was completed to that standard of reliability.

5. Affiliation motivation was assessed using the Thematic Apperception Test (TAT) for which participants wrote stories in response to several ambiguous picture stimuli. All coding was completed blind to year and all other data, using Winter's (1991) running-text coding system, by coders achieving and maintaining a reliability standard of at least .85 with expert scoring.

6. All coding took place with interviews from the 2 years mixed together. Coders were required to attain .85 interrater reliability at the beginning of the coding process, and systematic double coding ensured that all of the coding was completed to that standard of reliability. Although interviews were rated on a 5-point scale, scores were collapsed to 3 points (high, medium, low) before aggregation.

7. Power motivation was assessed using the TAT for which subjects wrote stories in response to several ambiguous picture stimuli. All coding was completed blind to year and all other data using Winter's (1991) running-text coding system by coders achieving and maintaining a reliability of at least .85 with expert scoring.

CHAPTER 6

Beyond the "Effects of Divorce on Children"
UNCOVERING AND UNDERSTANDING COMPLEXITY

For adults, the answer to the question "What helped people feel better?" changed with time. Early on, those elements useful in setting up new routines and establishing new household rules were related to better adjustment. A year later, the salient features were whatever was useful in setting up and maintaining relationships with other people. We asked the same question for children and came up with an answer that did not change much over time. For children, "what helped" was pretty much the same both years, perhaps because divorce, for most of the children in our sample, represented fundamentally an emotional, not a practical, challenge. That is, from the beginning of *children's* awareness, parents were taking care of the practical concerns and could only move on to relationship concerns with time. The children's task, on the other hand, was primarily the emotional one of dealing with a change in their family and household relationships. Their task stayed this way across the time of our study.

We found that during this period children's adjustment was rarely a simple function of their sex, age, or family circumstance. Far more often, their adjustment depended on how their level of understanding meshed with the challenges they faced, particularly the salience for them of their parents' distress. Specifically, we found that having mature social cognitive skills was generally helpful for children in potentially challenging situations but was

This chapter was drafted by Anne P. Copeland.

unrelated to (or actually a liability for) the adjustment of children in less challenging ones. Similarly, the importance of peer and sibling relationships depended on the children's family circumstance. In some cases, being involved with peers outside the household was related to better adjustment; in other cases, involvement with siblings was more predictive of good adjustment. The ways in which children's individual characteristics interacted with their family situations in affecting their adjustment is the focus of this chapter.

MEASURING CHILDREN'S ADJUSTMENT

The adjustment measures we have focused on have already been described in Chapter 2: children's psychological adjustment, illness, and behavior problems as rated by mothers and teachers. As expected, these four measures were related to each other, especially at Time 1. For example, children with good psychological adjustment tended to have few behavior problems. However, physical illness was not related to behavior problems (see Appendix Table 6.1).

Our working assumption was that it was better for a child to have higher scores on psychological adjustment and lower ones on illness and behavior problems at both Times 1 and 2. We recognize that this, in fact, may not be true. It is possible, for example, that children who have an immediate strong negative reaction to parental separation (as might be measured by low levels of self-reported psychological adjustment or lots of behavior problems) might be effectively expressing their anger or distress in ways that facilitate later, more permanent, better adjustment. Our analysis strategy would allow this result to be revealed, but in terms of predictions, we felt it was more sensible to work under the assumption that "better adjustment scores are better."

Second, we treated the four adjustment measures as four facets of the same global construct. We did not make specific predictions about each adjustment measure. Instead, we considered our measurement strategy one of getting reports about a range of types of adjustment from a variety of reporters.

We were able to compare the adjustment of the children in our sample with those in normative studies that had used the same form of three measures: the mother- and teacher-reported behavior problems measures (CBCL) and one of the components of the psychological adjustment measure, Harter's (1982) perceived competence ratings. Our sample's mean scores for mother-reported behavior problems (shown in Appendix Table 6.2) ranged from 32 to 42 at Time 1 and from 26 to 34 at Time 2, with standard deviations around 20. Not surprisingly, given that all of our children were in the throes of a recent parental separation, these scores are higher than the mean scores reported by Achenbach, Verhulst, Baron and Althaus (1987) in normative studies of children age 6–11 (the mean was about 20). But 67% of our girls and 45% of our boys at Time 1 were still below the cutoff points (set at 37 for girls and 40 for boys at this age) that Achenbach and Edelbrock (1981) recommended as useful for diagnostic purposes. By Time 2, 75% of the girls and 67% of the boys were below the cutoff point. This means that most of the children's scores were within the normal range.

The fact that the mothers who were rating children's behavior were also going through a stressful period may have affected their judgments of the children's behavior problems. This possibility is suggested by the fact that the teacher ratings on the CBCL were consistently as low as or lower than the scores reported by Edelbrock and Achenbach (1984) for their nonclinical sample of 150 6- to 8-year-olds (average total raw score was about 23) and 150 9- to 11-year-olds (average raw score about 22). (The children's scores in the various age/gender groups in our sample averaged between 4 and 17.)

On the Harter Perceived Competence Scale, the average raw subscale scores for cognitive and social competence and for general self-worth ranged from 2.8 to 3.2 for the four age and gender groups, as did the means in four normative samples reported by Harter (1982). Standard deviations (between 0.50 and 0.70) were also equivalent.

Thus, our sample was similar to children in normative samples in self-perceived competence, and in behavior problems as reported by teachers. Mothers' reports of behavior problems were somewhat higher than the levels of nonclinical samples, although most of our sample fell in the nonclinical range, especially by Time 2.

THE CONTEXTS OF CHILDREN'S ADJUSTMENT

In addition to looking at sex and age differences over time, we used three different kinds of factors in trying to understand how children differed in adjustment. First, as we did with adults, we assessed a variety of household characteristics that the literature on and folklore about divorce suggested might affect adjustment. Are children with highly conflictual parents more at risk? Does having a mother who is employed full-time affect reaction to divorce? Do children undergoing concomitant changes in their living situations do less well?

Second, we examined the role of peer support in children's adjustment. Does interaction with friends help? How about time spent with siblings, who are going through the same process?

And finally, we looked at a number of aspects of children's individual development, thinking that these might be directly related to children's adjustment. Children, in contrast with adults, were expected to differ in how well they understood what was going on in the course of parental separation. So we examined whether children who were more able to take another person's perspective in understanding a situation, or who had a more differentiated view of people, would have better adjustment. And we asked whether those who were less (or perhaps more) self-conscious, or who had a stronger sense of personal control over events, would be better adjusted.

However, we knew that it was likely that these individual and situational factors would be related to adjustment for some children but not others, and we wanted to refine these predictions. We thought it unlikely that particular kinds of children would always do well in responding to divorce, or that particular situations would always be trying. Rather, it seemed more likely that some situations would be more stressful for some people than others, and/or would call on different kinds of individual strengths. Further, it seemed likely that some personal characteristics would be helpful under some conditions but get in the way in others.

These, then, are the overarching questions examined in this chapter:

1. Do boys and girls, and younger (6- to 8-year-old) and older (9- to 12-year-old) children, differ in adjustment at Time 1 and Time 2? Do boys have a harder time, as many have suggested? Do girls reveal stress differently than boys?
2. Is the nature of the household directly related to adjustment? Specifically, do children have a harder adjustment if they have recently undergone many changes along with parental divorce, have working mothers, and/or have highly conflictual parents?
3. Is adjustment easier for children if they spend more time with peers and siblings?
4. Is a child's ability to think complexly about social situations (individual social-cognitive maturity) a direct benefit to adjustment?
5. Are individual characteristics differentially important in various postseparation situations?

DO BOYS AND GIRLS, AND YOUNGER AND OLDER CHILDREN, DIFFER IN ADJUSTMENT?

First, the simple findings (see Appendix Tables 6.2a–d): Across time, older and younger children did not differ from each other in how adjusted they seemed, even when we compared older and younger boys versus girls. And we found only two simple sex differences: (1) Girls were reported (by their mothers) to have more illnesses than boys and (2) teachers described boys as having more behavior problems than girls. Because we do not have a comparison group of children with nondivorcing parents, we cannot know for sure whether this means that girls tend to respond to divorce by being ill and boys by acting up at school, or whether these sex differences merely reflect sex differences that are commonly found in the general population.

We found three different answers to our question, "did over-time changes in adjustment differ for the sexes and age groups?" These results are presented against the backdrop of significant Time 1–Time 2 improvements in all adjustment measures except illness, for all the age–sex groups combined. Examining the age groups separately, older children at Time 2 were found to have better psychological adjustment compared to their own scores at Time 1 and compared to the younger group at either Time.[1] Perhaps older children can "bounce back" psychologically more quickly than younger children. Or, it could be that older children had suffered relatively greater losses in adjustment at Time 1, from which they recovered particularly well by Time 2.

Second, younger children were found to have better health than older children at Time 2 and better health than they themselves had had at Time 1.[2] Maybe these older children (who, we just learned, had better psychological well-being at Time 2) were nevertheless not feeling better physically. Or, it may be that younger children's greater "resilience," or ability to "bounce back," was in the domain of physical health.

And finally, boys at Time 1 were rated by their teachers as having more behavior problems than were girls, and more than either boys or girls at Time 2.[3] Again, however, we cannot know for sure whether these are findings about postdivorce adjustment or about development per se. Still, the findings are consistent with an interpretation about divorce that boys tended to respond in the immediate postseparation period with behavior problems.

Generally, then, our findings suggest that, over time, the children showed improved adjustment. The findings do not support the often-cited notion that boys had a harder time with divorce than girls. Although boys were described by their teachers as having more behavior problems (especially in the first 6 months), girls were seen by their mothers as having more illnesses. And while these may both be indicators of some kind of distress, we can't be sure of this because we know that, regardless of divorce, boys in general are reported to have more "externalizing" (behavioral) problems than girls and girls to have more "internalizing" (depression or anxiety) problems than boys (Achenbach & Edelbrock, 1978; Achenbach et al., 1987). Finally, we cannot conclude, as others have, that divorce is harder for one age group than another. In our study, the experience was different (but not harder) for different groups: Older children showed improvements in their psychological adjustment over time and younger children, in their physical well-being. (See Kalter, 1990, for an excellent account of age differences in children's reactions across a wider age range.)

IS THE NATURE OF THE HOUSEHOLD
DIRECTLY RELATED TO ADJUSTMENT?

We wanted to examine the direct effect that various postseparation household situations might have on children. In most cases, these were situations that were also examined with respect to adults' adjustment. We added one other—number of postseparation changes—that is often assumed to be especially important for children's adjustment. (The role of fathers' visitation—another important issue for children—is discussed in Chapter 10.) We considered the following:

- *Mother's work status* (coded from her interviews for whether she had paid employment on a full-time basis, or not).
- *Number of postseparation changes the child encountered* (coded from mothers' interviews for such things as whether the child started a new school or moved to a new home).
- *Parental conflict* (a combined score including level of postseparation interpersonal conflict between parents, referred to in Chapter 5, plus the number of court-filed motions by either member of the couple concerning the divorce, discussed in Chapter 8).

We examined whether any of these three postseparation household situations was correlated with any of the adjustment measures, separately at Time 1 and Time 2. A few modest direct relationships were found (see Appendix Table 6.3). At Time 1, the more mothers worked, the fewer behavior problems they said their children had. The more parent conflict existed, the more behavior problems both the mother and teacher reported for the child. Number of recent changes was not directly related to any child adjustment measure. Our conclusion was that, even though there was some support for the relevance of these variables, by themselves they told us very little about what children's adjustment was likely to be.

WHAT ROLE DOES PEER SUPPORT
PLAY FOR CHILDREN?

In the course of the children's interviews, we asked about their weekly schedules and activities. These sections of the interview were coded for *number of activities* typically engaged in with *siblings* and with *friends*.[4] Neither measure—activities with siblings nor friends—was directly related to children's adjustment (see Appendix Table 6.4).

ARE CHILDREN'S WAYS OF UNDERSTANDING DIRECTLY RELATED TO THEIR ADJUSTMENT?

Like adults, children have individual characteristics or traits that might be expected to be related to their adjustment to parental divorce. In addition, however, children's views of their families, more than adults', are colored by their developmental ability. We might expect younger or less mature children to be less adept at understanding the complexities of interpersonal relationships than older or more mature children. We might expect the children's degree of self-consciousness to be related to their adjustment. And perhaps more instrumental children—those who believe that they can take action in the world that will be helpful to them—will have better adjustment. In short, it seemed important to understand how children apply their cognitive, or thinking, abilities to the arena of social relationships. Can they understand that others might have a different reaction to the divorce than they have? Do they view others in a complex, multidimensional way, or are others seen as simply "good" or "bad"? Although adults may differ in these abilities as well, children's social-cognitive level is likely to vary significantly as a function of their age and maturity, and so seemed particularly important to capture.

We measured these individual characteristics from a variety of data sources about the child's individual psychological make-up, including children's interview responses and questionnaire data. It is important to note that, because we did not gather any data before the separation, we cannot know for sure whether these scores describe what the children were like prior to the separation, or whether they, instead, capture what they were like afterward, including any changes they may have undergone as a result of the separation. Our focus must remain squarely on the postseparation period, and the factors that coincide with current adjustment. Here is a list of the developmental measures we included:

1. *Perspective-taking ability* involved coding how well the child could describe the reactions of other family members to the separation and the feelings of other family members toward other aspects of their lives, using a modification of an approach originally derived for assessing perspective taking from interviews about family relationships and intimacy (White, Speisman, & Costos, 1983; White, Speisman, Jackson, Bartis, & Costos, 1986). Interviews were coded on 8-point scales, ranging from

- No recognition of perspectives other than one's own, to
- Recognition but rejection of other perspectives, to
- Recognition of alternative viewpoints and an awareness that different perspectives are a function both of internal needs, motives, and feel-

ings of the other person and of the interactive quality of relationships.

A child with a very low level of perspective taking assumes that different
members of a relationship share the same perspective. For example, one boy
responded to the question, "Why does your mother yell at you?" by saying,
"To aggravate me." A moderate, but somewhat egocentric level of perspective
taking would be reflected when children can represent the other's perspective
vis-à-vis him/herself, but cannot understand less directly self-relevant aspects
of the other's perspective. For example, one older child said, "My father used
to get upset when I would fool around in school. I can't blame him. If I had a
kid and he got in trouble in school I would be upset too." Full perspective taking is reflected when children can see things through others' eyes. In discussing his sister's response to the divorce, one boy said he thought his sister
was more bothered than he was. He indicated that this was because "my sister
used to be, like, my father's pet, so he's a god to her. She always looks up to
him." Here the child understands the reason for his sister's distress in terms of
her relationship with her father, and without reference to his own feelings or
relationships.

2. *Person-conception ability* involved coding the child's complexity of
person concepts in terms of the kinds of attributes used to describe others
(e.g., dispositional vs. physical) and the degree of egocentrism reflected in the
description (Peevers & Secord, 1973). Specifically, the coding system provides
three scores for each attribute ascribed to a family member:

a. Descriptiveness, or the degree to which the attribute differentiates the
person described from others.
b. Depth, or the degree to which the attribute reflects a superficial versus insightful description.
c. Involvement, or the degree of egocentrism reflected in the description.

Children who had relatively simple person concepts described their mothers
in terms such as, "I like everything about her," "She's nice," or "She brings us
places." Children with more complex person concepts described their mothers in ways like, "She's understanding with us because she knows we miss my
dad," or "Sometimes she takes us places even though she's tired and I know
she doesn't really feel like it."

3. *Self-consciousness* refers to a child's tendency to feel uncomfortable in
social situations because of a high degree of self-awareness. Self-consciousness reflects both an ability to imagine how others see oneself, and a tendency
to view others as potentially critical or judgmental. We used the Rosenberg
(1965) Self-Consciousness Scale, which children answered orally during the

interview. Children answered questions such as, "Do you get nervous when you're with people because you worry about how much they like you? (often, sometimes, or never)," and "Let's say some grownup or adult visitor came into class and the teacher wanted him to know who you were, so she asked you to stand up and tell the visitor a little about yourself. Would you like that, or would you not like that, or wouldn't you care?" We anticipated that, although self-consciousness reflects more advanced cognitive processes than its absence, children who were more self-conscious would find parental separation more difficult to adapt to than children who were less self-conscious.

4. The children's *locus of control*, or sense that they are in control of what happens in life, especially in terms of whether their cognitive abilities will serve them well, was also assessed orally, by presenting items from the Intellectual Achievement Responsibility Scale (Crandall, Katkovsky, & Crandall, 1965). Scores presented here reflect children's assessment of the degree to which they were in control of their success experiences. For example, children who report that if they do well on an exam, it is because they studied hard would be scored in the "internal" direction. Children who report that if they did well on an exam it would be because they were lucky, or the exam was easy, would be scored in the "external" direction.

We examined whether these individual characteristics—perspective taking, person conception, self-consciousness, and locus of control—were related to children's adjustment by looking at the correlations among the measures, separately for Time 1 and Time 2. (We first established that any relationships between ways of understanding and children's adjustment were not simply due to children's verbal intelligence.[5]) Table 6.1 and Appendix Table 6.5 summarize the findings.

All of these results are modestly in the direction predicted by the clinical and developmental literature and serve to give us some broad notions of what the helpful individual characteristics are for adjustment (to divorce or perhaps simply within the general population). Being less self-conscious was

TABLE 6.1. Relationships between Children's Adjustment and Developmental Characteristics

This adjustment measure:	Better psychological adjustment	More physical illness	More behavior problems—mother	More behavior problems—teacher
Was related to Time 1:	Lower self-consciousness	Less mature person concepts	Higher self-consciousness	External locus of control
Was related to Time 2:	Lower self-consciousness			

related to better self-reported adjustment at both times, and to fewer mother-reported behavior problems at Time 1. Also at Time 1, being less mature in person-concept ability was related to more mother-reported illnesses, and being external in locus of control was related to more teacher reports of behavior problems. Findings were stronger in the analyses within Time 1, suggesting that these individual vulnerabilities and strengths made the most difference to children's adjustment immediately following the separation, and faded in their significance with time.

ARE INDIVIDUAL AND PEER SUPPORT CHARACTERISTICS DIFFERENTIALLY IMPORTANT?

This question was addressed by using the data sources already described—the measures of adjustment, the measures of postseparation household situations, the measures of peer support, and the individual characteristics—now all together in a series of analyses (multiple regressions) that could consider three domains simultaneously.[6] In each analysis, we asked whether one individual trait (e.g., locus of control) or peer support measure (e.g., activities with friends) was more or less important for children in each postseparation household situation (e.g., mothers employed vs. not employed). For each household situation, we report findings concerning the individual traits, then the peer support measures. Because we were interested in fine-grained complexities here, we did this set of regressions for each Time, and for the total sample and boys and girls separately. The only findings reported here are ones in which the individual or peer support characteristic meant one thing in one postseparation household situation and had a different meaning (or was not related) in another postseparation situation.[7]

Several comments will serve to orient the reader. First, this account is based on within-Time 1 analyses. Results from over time or within-Time 2 analyses are reported when they bolster *or* when they differ in enlightening ways from the findings from within Time 1. Mostly, however, the results for children did not indicate changes in the pattern of relationships, as the results for adults did. Instead, mostly what was true at Time 1 was true at Time 2, and other factors served to differentiate children's adjustment. Gender differences were consistently important in some analyses—where this was true, results from the total sample (boys and girls analyzed together) are not reported.

Dealing with Parental Conflict

Because it is so central to the divorce situation, children's reactions to parental conflict are discussed in depth in Chapter 8. Here we examine only the ways in which individual developmental characteristics of children were useful, or not useful, in dealing with parental conflict. We thought that children with stronger skills at interpersonal understanding would be able to handle the more stressful situation of having parents in open conflict, but we weren't so sure those skills would matter much for children in low-conflict families. We thought of this as the "challenge hypothesis," figuring that under challenging conditions, individual skills would be more needed and thus more powerful predictors of adjustment, whereas in the less challenging situation, a wider range of individual characteristics might lead to good adjustment.

As predicted, adjustment of children with more conflictual parents (at both Times 1 and 2) was related more consistently to Time 1 individual developmental measures than was the adjustment of children with less conflictual parents. The results are summarized in Table 6.2 and Appendix Table 6.6.

Table 6.2 shows that if children with highly conflictual parents had more mature perspective-taking abilities, they had better psychological adjustment at both Times 1 and 2. Similarly, if children with highly conflictual parents had a more internal locus of control at Time 1, they tended to have better ad-

TABLE 6.2. Relationships between Times 1 and 2 Developmental Characteristics and Times 1 and 2 Adjustment of Children with Highly Conflictual Parents

	Mature perspective taking		Mature person concepts		Internal locus of control		Low self-consciousness		Sibling activities		Friend activities	
	T1	T2	T1	T2	T1	T2	T1	T2	T1	T2	T1	T2
T1 Psychological adjustment	+				+							
T2 Psychological adjustment	+				+							
T1 Illness			− (g)		−				+			
T2 Illness												
T1 Behavior problems—mother					−							
T2 Behavior problems—mother												
T1 Behavior problems—teacher			− (b)		−						−	
T2 Behavior problems—teacher												

Note. + indicates that scores were significantly positively related; − indicates that scores were significantly negatively related; (g) indicates "for girls only" and (b) "for boys only."

justment (better psychological adjustment, less illness, fewer behavior problems) at Time 1. They also had better psychological adjustment at Time 2. And, finally, these children had better adjustment (measured differently for boys and girls) at Time 1 if, at Time 1, they had more differentiated person-concept skills.[8] No relationships among parental conflict, individual developmental characteristics, and adjustment were significant within Time 2. Thus, it seems that having social-cognitive skills to call on in the immediate post-separation period was adaptive, both concurrently and a year later, for children with highly conflictual parents. One boy revealed the complexity of his perceptions, in describing how his parents got along after the separation, and in particular, referring to a recent family graduation party: "It can be very good and it can be very bad, depends. Most of the time at the party they got along very well; it just happened that one incident, they didn't. It was perfect except for that."

The adjustment of children in families with less conflictual parents was either unrelated to these measures (as predicted) or, in a few cases, was related in the opposite way. Specifically, children whose parents were low in conflict had *lower* psychological adjustment scores (at both Times 1 and 2) if they had better perspective-taking abilities and more internal locus of control; this pattern was not found within Time 2. It may have been that, because their parents were not overtly conflictual, these children who were perceptive and instrumental were confused about the separation and perhaps felt some degree of responsibility for it, lowering their psychological adjustment scores. For example, one girl, whose parents scored low on conflict, had witnessed little or no fighting between her parents before the separation. Nevertheless, she had been told by them that they had been fighting a lot prior to the separation. When asked how she thought her mother felt about being separated, she told us, "Well, before they got divorced I know they were fighting a lot. I know she doesn't like to fight, so I think she probably is glad that she doesn't have to fight anymore." It seems clear that this child is struggling to use the information she's been given (that they were fighting) and to square it with what she "knows" from her experience to be true (that they do not fight). Being more perceptive in this case makes the task of accepting her parents' account of the causes of the separation more difficult for her.

The meaning of social support also differed for the highly and less-conflictual groups. At Time 1, children with parents in conflict were better adjusted (as indicated by having fewer illnesses) if they did fewer activities with their siblings. Their adjustment (as indicated by fewer teacher-rated behavior problems) was better if they were more involved in activities with their friends. The opposite was true of children with parents low in conflict—they were better adjusted if they pursued more activities with their siblings and fewer activities with their friends.

In short, children tended to benefit from family/sibling-centered activity if the parents were getting along, and from outside-the-family activity if the parents were conflictual. For example, one child, whose parents had very high levels of conflict, said she didn't talk about the divorce with her siblings: "None of us want to really talk about it to anyone in the family because they might feel differently . . . we just talk to our friends about it." Another child with highly conflictual parents found help outside the family: "I didn't know how to do [my homework] 'cause the teacher explained it when I was absent. The teacher said we'd be in big trouble if we didn't do it, so I didn't know how to do it, so I went next door to our friend—she's 18 or 19—and she helped me."

In contrast, a girl whose parents scored low in conflict described turning to her younger brother when upset: "I can tell him something real important—secrets—and he won't tell." There seemed to be a latent positive effect for these children, however, of doing lots of activities with friends immediately after the separation; by Time 2, those who had spent more time with friends right after the separation were better adjusted. Thus, while staying family focused in the early postseparation days was helpful at the time to children in low-conflict families, time spent with friends turned out to have been a positive step for them by Time 2. This result parallels results for mothers, for whom emotional support in the immediate postseparation period only paid off with better adjustment at Time 2.

Mothers' Work Status

We examined the meaning of mothers' employment status next. Our assumption was that having a mother who works full-time would have both costs and benefits for children, as would having a mother who did not work outside the home as much or at all. Employed mothers, for example, may be able to provide more material resources, they may have better psychological adjustment themselves (as our results in Chapter 5 suggest), and, in being around less, may cause the child to be exposed to more extrafamilial experiences that may provide a distraction from thinking about the divorce. Mothers who are employed part-time or not at all, in contrast, may be more available to their children as psychological resources, although they may also indirectly remind their children of the divorce or more directly expose them to their own distress. These situations may call on different strengths from children in order to adjust optimally, so we carefully examined interactions between work status and children's individual characteristics. The overall findings supported our conclusion that maternal employment did not play a simple role in children's adjustment; it was unrelated to three of the indicators, and positively related only to mothers' reports of children's behavior (with employed mothers reporting fewer behavior problems).

Boys

Let us turn first to sons of mothers who were employed full-time. The results from this analysis, presented in Table 6.3 and Appendix Table 6.7, show that for boys with employed mothers, more internal locus of control was related to better psychological adjustment and less illness. Better perspective-taking skills were related to better psychological and behavioral adjustment but also to more illness. These personal characteristics led them, perhaps, to understand their families better and to respond to the autonomy and responsibility demands required of them by their mothers' employment status by overtly "pulling themselves together." One 7-year-old boy whose mother worked full-time, for example, seemed to be able to use his perceptiveness to understand his mother. At Time 2 he told us, "My mother seems a little bit happier, now that she can go out on a date and not have someone worry about it. . . . My father has a very special girlfriend. She said we could make doughnuts at home. I told my mother and I think she got a little jealous and that might've made her a little mad." This kind of perceptiveness may have had some cost, however, if we consider higher levels of illness to be an indicator of stress—in being so understanding and sympathetic, and

TABLE 6.3. Relationships between Times 1 and 2 Individual Characteristics and Times 1 and 2 Adjustment for Sons of Mothers Employed Full-Time

	Mature perspective taking		Mature person concepts		Internal locus of control		Self-consciousness	
	T1	T2	T1	T2	T1	T2	T1	T2
T1 Psychological adjustment	+							
T2 Psychological adjustment	+					+		
T1 Illness	+							
T2 Illness	+		+		−			
T1 Behavior problems—mother	−							
T2 Behavior problems—mother	−			+				
T1 Behavior problems—teacher								
T2 Behavior problems—teacher	−							

Note. + and − signs as in Table 6.2.

taking on so much autonomy, boys in this situation appeared to get sick more often.

A very different picture emerged for sons of mothers who worked part-time or less, as summarized in Table 6.4. Here, it seems that boys with mothers not employed full-time who have good perspective- taking skills and are highly self-conscious feel more overtly distressed, perhaps because they are in more direct and perceptive contact with their mothers' distress. One such child answered our question about how his mother felt about being separated this way:

> "I'd say she feels not so happy. . . . She hasn't got a job, so my father's paying her alimony. . . . She's gotta go out and make her own income, so, she doesn't feel happy about that. After a year, you know, she's gonna have to go out and get her own income from now on."

This direct expression of distress, as indicated by worse psychological adjustment and more behavior problems, however, may help free them from more internalized distress, as marked by illness levels.

TABLE 6.4. Relationships between Times 1 and 2 Individual Characteristics and Times 1 and 2 Adjustment for Sons of Mothers Not Employed Full-Time

	Mature perspective taking		Mature person concepts		Internal locus of control		Self-consciousness	
	T1	T2	T1	T2	T1	T2	T1	T2
T1 Psychological adjustment	−							
T2 Psychological adjustment	−							
T1 Illness	−							
T2 Illness	−							
T1 Behavior problems—mother	+							
T2 Behavior problems—mother	+			−			+	
T1 Behavior problems—teacher								
T2 Behavior problems—teacher							+	

Note. + and − signs as in Table 6.2.

Girls

The developmental factors did not significantly interact with mothers' work status for girls at all within Time 1 (see Appendix Table 6.8). This is quite interesting in itself. The same-sex parent–child relationship may somehow be important in making mothers' work status less important for girls, early on. Perhaps the demands on daughters who have mothers employed full-time and those who have mothers working less are more similar than they are for boys. This could result in daughters either feeling less responsibility or autonomy demand from employed mothers than boys do, or being less involved with or bothered by being with their mothers who are not employed full-time, compared with boys, or both.

But by Time 2, things changed. Table 6.5 shows the results for the daughters of mothers employed full-time. Table 6.6 shows the results for daughters of mothers who were not employed full-time.

In short, at Time 2 daughters of mothers who were employed full-time showed better psychological and behavioral adjustment (but more illness) if they had better perspective-taking abilities, more internal locus of control, and higher self-consciousness. The opposite was true for the part-time-work-

TABLE 6.5. Relationships between Times 1 and 2 Individual Characteristics and Times 1 and 2 Adjustment for Daughters of Mothers Employed Full-Time

	Mature perspective taking		Mature person concepts		Internal locus of control		Self-consciousness	
	T1	T2	T1	T2	T1	T2	T1	T2
T1 Psychological adjustment								
T2 Psychological adjustment	+					+		+
T1 Illness								
T2 Illness						+		
T1 Behavior problems—mother								
T2 Behavior problems—mother								−
T1 Behavior problems—teacher								
T2 Behavior problems—teacher								

Note. + and − signs as in Table 6.2.

TABLE 6.6. Relationships between Times 1 and 2 Individual Characteristics and Times 1 and 2 Adjustment for Daughters of Mothers Not Employed Full-Time

	Mature perspective taking		Mature person concepts		Internal locus of control		Self-consciousness		Sibling activities		Friend activities	
	T1	T2	T1	T2	T1	T2	T1	T2	T1	T2	T1	T2
T1 Psychological adjustment									+			
T2 Psychological adjustment	−				−			−	+	+	+	+
T1 Illness												
T2 Illness					−				−		−	−
T1 Behavior problems—mother											−	
T2 Behavior problems—mother								+				
T1 Behavior problems—teacher												
T2 Behavior problems—teacher				+	+		+			−		

Note. + and − signs as in Table 6.2.

or-less group—daughters with better perspective-taking abilities, more internal locus of control, and higher self-consciousness had worse adjustment on the same measures (and, in addition, had more behavior problems, according to their teachers).

Thus, by Time 2, when mothers were employed full-time and not around as much, girls with those characteristics having to do with sensitivity to others—like a more sophisticated understanding of people and more self-consciousness—seemed to do better, perhaps because their mothers were, in fact, themselves better adjusted, or perhaps because the daughters were not being confronted daily with stressed, worrisome mothers. One girl described what she liked about her mother, who was employed full-time: "She doesn't yell very often except when she's tired. She gets all cranky, but she doesn't yell. Sometimes if you're busy doing something and you ask her to get something for you, she'll do that."

In contrast, when the mothers who were not employed full-time were around more, these same characteristics were related to worse adjustment in their daughters—again, perhaps through their being confronted with their mothers' distress. For example, one daughter of a mother who was not employed full-time scored high (in the mature direction) on every one of our developmental measures and poorly in adjustment. In answering a question about what her mother was like, she told us, "She's nice, like, generous, but she can be real obnoxious too. Like, if she's in a bad mood and you ask her for something she'll scream and, like, blame it on you, take it out on me, whatever she's mad at." Being so tuned in to her mother apparently made this girl's adjustment more difficult.

Finally, for girls, whether social support was related to adjustment depended consistently on whether mothers were employed full-time or not, but did not matter consistently for boys.[9] For daughters of mothers not employed full-time, more activities with friends and siblings were related to better adjustment (as measured by all four adjustment measures), as assessed within Time 1, within Time 2, and across time. These activities may have helped distract these girls from their mothers' situation.

Summary of Findings about Mothers' Work Status

For both boys and girls, then, mature social-cognitive skills and an internal locus of control were eventually helpful to those with full-time employed mothers and actually unhelpful to those whose mothers were not employed full-time outside the home (though this was only true for girls by Time 2, not at Time 1). Having a more complex and sophisticated understanding of those around them was adaptive for children whose mothers were employed full-time and who perhaps had to "figure things out for themselves" more often. These same skills were not helpful to children of mothers who worked less than full-time (who we know may, in fact, have been more distressed than mothers who worked full-time). High levels of self-consciousness were particularly troublesome for this latter group. Perhaps in spending more time with a distressed mother, the more perceptive and self-focused children were too often faced with a difficult social relationship they could not really understand.

Finally, it is interesting to note that activities with siblings and friends were related to better adjustment more consistently for girls with mothers who were not employed full-time than for any other group. It may be that girls, more than boys, are able to use these social connections to aid their adjustment and to broaden their experience away from their available, but, as we saw in Chapter 5, more distressed mothers.

Facing Recent Changes

The meaning of encountering more changes (of school, residence, etc.) along with parental separation was different for boys and girls (see Appendix Tables

6.9 and 6.10, respectively). Boys encountering a lot of changes at the time of the separation had worse psychological and behavioral adjustment (at both Times 1 and 2) if they had better perspective-taking skills; the reverse was true for boys encountering fewer changes. Perhaps facing a larger number of changes is harder for boys who have better social-cognitive skills, precisely because the complexity of the task of adjustment is increased by their own level of understanding. For boys facing a simpler situation, perspective-taking skills were apparently useful and did not make the situation more overwhelming. One boy told us:

> "[The separation] really doesn't bother me that much 'cause nothing's really changed that much besides the house being a little happier. But, I mean, my father comes to basketball, softball games, or anything that I have, and like it's really seeing him the same, not as much, but . . . like, you can call him if something's wrong because we always know where he's going to be."

The opposite was true for girls, though only at Time 2—girls who had encountered a lot of postseparation changes had better behavioral adjustment if they also had better perspective-taking skills, more mature person concepts, and a more internal locus of control. That is, their social-cognitive skills aided their longer-term adjustment under conditions of more changes. These same girls also had better behavioral adjustment (at both Times 1 and Time 2) if they had higher self-consciousness scores (at either Time 1 or 2). The opposite was true of girls in more stable situations. One suggestion based on these results, coupled with the findings about girls' self-consciousness reported in the maternal work status section earlier, is that, contrary to our findings for the sample overall, low self-consciousness may not be the most adaptive stance for girls whose parents have recently separated. Perhaps for girls self-consciousness is an indicator of social skills and understanding, more than an inappropriate self-focus in social situations.

Peer support measures were not related to postseparation changes and adjustment in any consistent or coherent way, for either boys or girls.

CONCLUSIONS

In this chapter, we took two approaches to understanding children's response to divorce. First, we looked for fairly simple effects. We asked whether children's adjustment was related in a direct manner to their age or sex, to individual developmental characteristics (like social-cognitive abilities), to time spent with peers, or to differences in their postseparation household situations (e.g., whether their parents had a conflictual relationship or whether they had a lot of other changes in their lives besides the departure of their father).

We found that, with a few exceptions, age and gender had little direct effect on adjustment within this time period and within the age range represented by this sample. For the sample as a whole, we found that social understanding skills were associated with better adjustment overall at Time 1, but not at Time 2. And we found that, for the most part, peer activities and household situational characteristics were not especially important overall, taken by themselves (though parental conflict was generally problematic and maternal employment, somewhat helpful). In short, it seems that children's adjustment to divorce is not simply a function of a few personal or situational factors.

Our second approach involved examining these predictors of adjustment together. We think the results from these analyses are more enlightening about children's responses to divorce in this time frame and age range. They suggest that particular personal characteristics did meaningfully predict adjustment for children in some situations but not in others, and that boys and girls sometimes differed in what personal characteristics were important.

We knew that parental conflict was associated with poorer adjustment in children overall and that better social-cognitive skills were associated with better adjustment. What is really more important, though, is the finding that children in families with high levels of parental conflict were better adjusted if they had more mature or sophisticated ways of understanding, but that this was not true for children in families with low levels of conflict. It appears that sophisticated social understanding helps children who are facing especially difficult situations, but may unnecessarily complicate situations for children in less difficult circumstances.

It is difficult to know, across all of the children in the sample, what full-time maternal employment signified. Having a mother who works full-time is not exactly more or less challenging than having a mother who works part-time or not at all, but it is a different situation, apparently drawing on different skills. For both boys and girls whose mothers were employed full-time, having better perspective-taking skills and an internal locus of control (and, for girls only, higher self-consciousness) was helpful, whereas these characteristics were unhelpful, or even a liability, to children whose mothers were not employed full time. These social-cognitive skills may have helped children whose mothers were employed full-time to solve more independently than other children the practical and other problems they faced. On the other hand, those same social-cognitive skills may have led children whose mothers were at home more to tune in to their mothers' distress in a way that compromised their own well-being.

Finally, girls encountering more postseparation changes with better social-cognitive abilities were better adjusted, while the opposite was true for boys. Along with the evidence that the adjustment of girls, but not of boys, with mothers at home more was facilitated by social involvements, this finding suggests that girls may be more likely than boys to use social relationships as a support in managing stressful circumstances. In short, although our data do not indicate simple sex differences in reaction to divorce, they do suggest that boys and girls use different skills and traits to help them adjust under different circumstances. It is also striking that these results are consistent with those presented in Chapter 5—with very different measures—that suggested that social relationships were generally more beneficial for women and more problematic for men in the postseparation period.

We feel that blanket prescriptions for children facing parental separation and divorce are not warranted by our data. For example, boys did not clearly adjust better or worse than girls. It was not always bad to be self-conscious. Having a mother who was employed full-time was neither a clear liability nor a clear asset to all children. In fact, even being perceptive and mature in understanding the divorce was not always helpful; for children whose parents were not overtly conflictual, or whose mothers were at home a great deal, these characteristics seemed to make adjustment more difficult. Parents in low-conflict situations or in families where the mothers are not employed full-time would do well to avoid leaning on a perceptive child's abilities in human understanding. Confiding in and seeking advice from a perceptive son or daughter in these conditions may strain the child's coping abilities.

On the other hand, these skills at social understanding were used to good ends by children in other kinds of situations—those where mothers were employed full-time and where parents were highly conflictual. While asking any child to become an adult-like confidante for a parent is probably ill-advised, our results suggest that children in these situations attempt to cope with and master the process of divorce at least partially by effectively using their developmental skills, and that parents should try to support this coping strategy.

NOTES

1. $p < .001$ comparing older children at Times 1 and 2; $p < .001$ comparing older children at Time 2 with younger children at Time 1; $p < .05$ comparing older children at Time 2 with younger children at Time 2.

2. $p < .05$ comparing younger and older children at Time 2; $p < .05$ comparing younger children at Times 1 and 2.

3. $p < .001$ comparing boys and girls at Time 1; $p < .001$ comparing boys at Time 1 with both boys and girls at Time 2.

4. All coding discussed in this chapter took place with interviews from the 2 years mixed together. Coders were required to attain .85 interrater reliability at the beginning of the

coding process, and systematic double coding ensured that all of the coding was completed to that standard of reliability.

5. To do this, we used a brief measure of verbal intelligence (the Vocabulary subscale score on the Wechsler Intelligence Scale for Children—Revised; Wechsler, 1974). Verbal intelligence was not significantly related to any of the four adjustment measures at either time. It was unrelated to Times 1 and 2 perspective-taking ability, person conception, and Time 2 self-consciousness. It was modestly but significantly related to Time 1 self-consciousness, $r = .23$, and Times 1 and 2 internal locus of control, $r = .26$ and .28, respectively. However, the significant relationships reported in this chapter (between ways of understanding and adjustment) remained after we controlled for the verbal intelligence score in the analysis.

6. In addition, multiple regression analyses helped preserve sample size.

7. In the text, all significant ($p < .05$) results from post hoc analyses of significant interaction terms are reported.

8. For girls, beta for interaction term predicting illness $= -1.97$, $t = -2.28$, $p < .05$; for boys, beta for interaction term predicting teacher-rated behavior problems $= -2.42$, $t = -2.15$, $p < .05$.

9. At Time 1, boys who had mothers employed less than full-time and who did more activities with friends had more behavior problems (as rated by mothers) at Time 1. At Time 2, these same boys had better psychological adjustment and more illness.

PART THREE

FAMILY DYADS, ADJUSTMENT, AND CHANGE

In this part we explore the mother–child dyad and the parent dyad. We consider how these dyads change over time, and how the relationships influence and reflect the adjustment of the individuals in them.

In Chapter 7, we explore the mother–child relationship in some detail. We found that mothers' and children's adjustment and the quality of their relationships were deeply interconnected, especially during the early period. We found, too, that how mothers' and children's other relationships were going affected their relationship with each other in the early period. In contrast, economic resources and the adjustment of other household members affected their relationship more later. Overall, this chapter confirms that the mothers' and children's well-being were intimately tied to their relationships with each other and suggests that this dyadic relationship is embedded in other important relationships too.

In Chapter 8, we examine the impact of parental conflict on children's well-being. Because it is well established that parental conflict is problematic for children, we attempt to identify the different kinds of conflict: physical violence, verbal conflict, legal conflict, and so forth. In addition, we examine the relationship between parents' adjustment and interparental conflict. These analyses make clear that different groups of children were affected differently by parental conflict and that mothers were somewhat affected by conflict too.

Because conflict is such a defining feature of divorce, and both children's and mothers' adjustment is affected by it, we explore in depth the factors that limit and contain parental conflict in Chapter 9. In this chapter, we examine interviews with 22 couples in which both members of the couples participated in the study at both times. We describe the many features that differentiate couples in which parents are in open, unconstrained conflict versus those who are "allies" and coparents. We also explore the features of couples less extreme in their postseparation conflict patterns.

Overall these three chapters underscore the links between the dyads examined and the well-being of family members outside that dyad. They naturally draw our attention to the family as a unit, which we will turn to in Part IV.

CHAPTER 7

The Mother–Child Relationship
INSIDER AND OUTSIDER VIEWS

So far in this book we have been examining how individuals proceed through the steps of divorce, focusing mainly on aspects of those individuals' lives that make things easier or harder. We have noticed that these processes are sometimes different for adults and children, and males and females. So what happens to *family relationships* across genders and generations during parental divorce? Can we learn more about individuals' adjustment if we understand the relationships in which they are embedded? Is a child's adjustment connected in some way to the adjustment of the parents and siblings? And is the mother's adjustment connected in a similar way? What makes for good family relationships in the first place? What are the contextual factors, both inside the family and outside, that affect adjustment? Can we begin to understand the intricate web of influence on individual adjustment by examining the relationships connecting individuals to others?

In this chapter, we will take a close look at the relationship between the mothers and children. There were too few father-custody families in our sample to conduct parallel analyses with them, but we do include attention to the meaning of the father–child relationship (as reported by family members) for children's adjustment. And we will bring the fathers back into full

This chapter was drafted by Anne P. Copeland.

view in the next two chapters when we turn to the mother–father relationship and the family as a whole.

The mother–child relationship has a long-standing and prized role in the field of psychology, especially for those interested in psychological development across the lifespan. Psychoanalysts, child developmentalists, and family theorists alike have written about how this bond has far-reaching implications. Those interested in children at risk—for emotional problems, behavior disorders, and cognitive deficits—also tend to pay at least some attention to the mother–child relationship.

Until quite recently, however, writing in this area has been marked by two limitations. First, almost exclusive attention has been paid to the meaning and outcome of the relationship for the *child* rather than the mother—that is, the questions of how best to provide day care, foster care, or in-hospital care, for example, have largely centered on the ramifications for the child of disruptions to the mother–child relationship. Much less attention has been paid to the role of the mother–child relationship in the *mother's* growth and identity. Whether having children, and having a good relationship with them, has an influence on women's adjustment, or their ability to cope with stress, for example, are questions that are much less common, though no less important.

A second limitation in our understanding stems from the assumption in much of the traditional writing about the mother–child pair that the meaning of the relationship (for the child) can and should be understood in simple cause-and-effect terms, that is, "How does the quality of the mother–child relationship affect the child?" What is ignored in this question is the possibility that qualities of the child and the mother—for example, their adjustment levels—may affect the relationship (instead of or in addition to the other way around), and that forces inside and outside the family have an ever-present bearing on the mother–child relationship.

In our approach to the study of the mother–child relationship following separation, we have tried to address these additional concerns by examining the evolving, reciprocal relationship, and how it affects and is affected by the family. We have included views of the family from nonfamily members as well, both to get an outsider's perspective and to compare that to the insiders/family members' views of their relationships. This chapter is organized around three questions:

1. Is mother–child relationship quality in fact related to the adjustment of both mothers and children?
2. Do other aspects of mothers' and children's family lives have a bearing on the mother–child relationship?
3. Are there broader family contextual factors that are related to relationship quality?

MOTHER–CHILD RELATIONSHIP QUALITY
AND ADJUSTMENT

Measurement of Relationship Quality

Our first concern was to develop a way to measure the quality of the mother–child relationship that was sensitive to important differences in style and insensitive to unimportant ones. We had two relevant data sources available: a videotaped observation of the mother and child playing together and a questionnaire that the mothers completed about their attitudes about and approach to raising this particular child. Thus, we had both an "outsider's" view (the observational measure) and an "insider's" view (the self-report measure of the relationship) (Olson, 1977).

The *observational/outsider's measure* of relationship quality was obtained from coding a 30-minute play session, in which the mother and child engaged in free play, built a tower while the child was blindfolded, and made an arts project together. In the coding system we used (Mash, Terdal, & Anderson, 1973), verbal and nonverbal interchanges between mother and child are coded. Every 15 seconds we would record both how the child had just responded to what the mother had just done, and how the mother had just responded to what the child had just done. Each response was put into one of several categories; for this chapter, we report on a summary code that captures mutual involvement in the play by the mother and child and the degree to which they were playing together either neutrally or positively.[1] Although all study families were invited to return for a second visit to participate in this portion of the study, only 62 families did so; thus, the sample for observational measures is smaller than in other chapters, making it impossible to examine possible subgroup differences among the children. The mothers and children of these 62 families did not differ from the sample as a whole, however, on any of the four child or two adult adjustment measures.

The *self-report/insider's measure* of relationship quality was taken from mothers' completion of Block's (1965) Childrearing Practices Report. We created a score combining mothers' enjoyment/warmth and their lack of a detached or negative control style. Examples of items on the enjoyment/warmth factor are the following:

- "I find some of my greatest satisfactions in my child."
- "I express affection by hugging, kissing, and holding my child."
- "I am easy-going and relaxed with my child."

Examples of the control style factor are the following:

- "I often feel angry with my child."
- "I let my child know how ashamed and disappointed I am when he/she misbehaves."
- "I expect my child to be grateful and appreciative for all the advantages he/she has."

Scores on the latter factor were reversed before combining them with the warmth factor, so that a high score would indicate a positive, less controlling relationship. Mothers completed this measure specifically in terms of their relationship with the focus child, and it was therefore felt to be an important, if indirect, indicator of the nature of their relationship. The self-report and observational measures were significantly correlated with each other, suggesting that insider and outsider views were not widely discrepant.

Measurement of Children's and Mothers' Adjustment

The four indicators of children's adjustment and two indicators of mothers' adjustment, already described in Chapter 2, were used to examine the meaning of relationship quality. First we asked whether mothers' adjustment and children's adjustment were related directly to each other. We examined boys and girls separately, but found that the patterns were very similar for the two groups, and clearer when the groups were combined (see Appendix Table 7.1 for a comparison of girls, boys, and the total sample). Specifically, we found that, at Time 1, mothers' own psychological adjustment was related to their ratings of their children's behavior problems. By Time 2, mothers' psychological adjustment was related to teachers' ratings of behavior problems as well. Mothers' self-reported psychological adjustment was not related to that of their children at either time. Mothers' reports of their own illness were related to their children's self-reported psychological adjustment (at Time 1 with the sexes combined, and for girls only, at Time 2 too). Mothers' illness ratings were also related to their own reports of their children's illness (at Time 2) and to their reports of their children's behavior problems at both times.

Clearly, with this pattern of results it would be simplistic to conclude that mothers who were better adjusted had better adjusted children. It is true that children's behavior problems, as reported by mothers, were consistently related to mothers' psychological adjustment and illness, but other indicators of children's adjustment were not consistently tied to mothers' adjustment. Several possibilities exist about the meaning of these interrelationships, and maybe all are true. It could be that children react to their mothers' strain with more behavior problems, but not more internalized kinds of stress. This interpretation is not supported by the finding that mothers with more illlness (a different kind of strain) had children with both higher externalizing (behavior problems) and internalizing (illness and psychological adjustment) problems.

Alternately, it could be that children who are behaving in a nonproblematic way help their mothers be better adjusted. Or it could be that mothers in distress describe their children as more troubled (even if they aren't). Only at Time 2, for example, did teacher reports of children's behavior problems correlate with mothers' adjustment. It is clear that mothers' and children's adjustment are linked, but in complex and interesting ways.

In this chapter we examine the possibility that both mothers' and children's adjustment are linked to the quality of the relationship they have with each other. We will keep these possibilities in mind throughout this chapter and will pay particular attention to how outsiders—like the teachers—see the family. That teachers and mothers tended to see the children the same way (see Chapter 6) gives us confidence that our various views of adjustment converge and are not simply a function of mothers' bias.

Analysis Strategy and Results

Using our standard measures of mother and child adjustment, and the measures of relationship quality, we asked the following questions,[2] as depicted in Figure 7.1:

- Is there a connection between relationship quality and adjustment in the immediate postseparation period?
- Is there a difference in the strength of this connection between relationship quality and adjustment a year later?
- Is relationship quality at Time 1 related to adjustment a year later?

Because of the smaller sample available for observational coding, we did not conduct these analyses separately for boys and girls. Appendix Table 7.2,

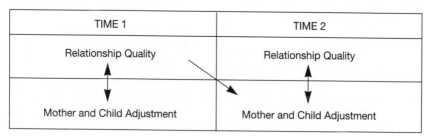

TIME 1	TIME 2
Relationship Quality	Relationship Quality
Mother and Child Adjustment	Mother and Child Adjustment

FIGURE 7.1. Analysis strategy: Links between relationship quality and child adjustment.

however, shows that the simple correlations between relationship quality and adjustment were generally similar for the two sexes.

Is there a connection between relationship quality and adjustment in the immediate postseparation period? At Time 1, the clear answer is "Yes," for both mothers and children. More specifically, the two measures of relationship quality (taken from the videotaped observation coding and from the mothers' questionnaire) were correlated with both children's psychological and behavioral adjustment levels (as reported by both mothers and teachers) and mothers' psychological adjustment levels. Relationship quality was not related to illness levels for either mothers or children (see Appendix Table 7.3).

It should be noted that our data do not allow us to make any clear claims about the direction of causality—whether having a better relationship with one's mother or child causes one to be better adjusted or whether being better adjusted allows one to have a better relationship cannot be determined with certainty.

We noticed one further interesting detail in the results concerning relationship quality and adjustment. The adjustment reports made by the two insiders involved (the mother and the child)—that is, the child and mother self-reports of adjustment and the mother rating of child behavior problems—were related to the maternal self-report questionnaire about relationship quality, which was the insider's account of the relationship. Interestingly, the outsider's view of the children's adjustment, that of the teacher, is the only adjustment measure that was significantly related to the observational measure—that is the outsider's account of the relationship—and the direction of the effect was surprising. Children with better observed relationship quality with their mothers were rated by their teachers as having more behavior problems. This finding is consistent with the notion that children in stress "hold it together" in some domains of their lives and "let it out" in others. It may also be that children whose behavior is problematic in school have more positive interactions in situations like this one, where they have lots of individual attention. It is possible, too, that these are children whose mothers have responded to their past distress by providing attentive support beyond the level the classroom teacher can offer.

When we reviewed the interviews and videotapes, the meaning of relationship quality scores became quite vivid. Interviews with the mothers who scored high on both of our mother–child relationship quality measures tended to be distinguished by continual, though often indirect, reference to the child as being an asset to the mother's life. Children were described as asking them interesting and thought-provoking questions, as asking to do activities that turned out to be fun for the mothers, or as presenting challenges that would be solved together. One child, for example, pressed his mother, at a time of distress, to go to the beach in the middle of winter; she reluctantly agreed, and she reported to us a memorable time, drinking hot chocolate and running along the shore. Another described her 7-year-old child's interests to be the same as hers: "She likes to read, she loves to write letters, she loves sports, which I think is great." In short, these mothers clearly saw themselves as "in the same boat" with their children.

In contrast, interviews with the mothers who scored low on both our relationship quality measures tended to present handling their children as one of their many problems. Less sense of connectedness and warmth came through. These interviews were not marked by any particular disdain or disregard for the children; few mothers said outright that they had "bad relationships" with their focus children, and few complained openly about caring for them. In fact, their surface descriptions were more likely to be positive, if fragile. For example, one mother with low relationship quality scores repeatedly asserted that her relationship with her son was "really getting a lot better." Underlying this characterization was a recent history of quite a negative relationship. More distinctive of this group was an aloofness, a separation of their concerns from their children's.

Differences in the observations between pairs with high and low relationship quality scores also seemed to revolve around involvement and empathy. Mothers and children with high scores tended to throw themselves into the free play, for example, making up stories for doll play with a shared theme, or making clay figures to tell a story together. These mothers were not just "willing participants" in their children's play, but rather made real suggestions that built on the play of the child and generally helped carry out the play themes. During the blindfolded tower-building task, these mothers were closely involved and interactive, making appropriate suggestions and generally being supportive. They reflected the child's affect, seeming genuinely pleased with tower-building success and lightly frustrated with falling blocks. It was a surprise to us, then, that these children were rated by their teachers as having more problems. The tone of the mother–child relationship seemed so genuinely positive in these pairs that we think the children expressed distress at school that they felt when they were away from the nurturing comfort of their mothers.

In contrast, low-scoring dyads were either quite aloof during the observations, with little interactive play, either verbally or behaviorally, or, in a few cases, actually negative in tone (characterized by sarcasm, criticism, and negative control strategies). During one such observation, for example, the mother was generally gruff and critical and laughed at her son's tower-building failures, despite his repeated request that she stop doing so. These children may have found school a respite from tense relationships at home, resulting in fewer reports of problems from teachers.

Is there a difference in the strength of the connection between relationship quality and adjustment a year later? We wanted to know whether having a good mother–child relationship continued to be related to adjustment at Time 2, or whether they were only related to each other during Time 1 (the period of maximum stress). We found that, within Time 2, relationship quality was significantly related only to the ratings of children's behavior problems by teachers and mothers in the same pattern as had been true within Time 1 (see Appendix Table 7.4). Relations to the psychological adjustment measures for both mothers and children disappeared, and, as had been true at Time 1, illness was not associated with relationship quality. The insider–outsider relationship was maintained, however; mothers' (insider) self-reports about their relationship continued to be significantly related to their (insider) ratings of their children, and observational (outsider) scores continued to be significantly related to the teacher (outsider) ratings. Thus, while the link between maternal reports about the relationship and maternal reports about the child's adjustment may be, at least in part, a function of reporter bias, outsiders to the system continue to confirm that the mother–child relationship and children's adjustment are connected to each other, even if in complex ways.

Again, it is important to keep in mind that no causality can be determined from these data. It is just as likely that children and mothers with better adjustment levels manage to develop a better relationship with each other as that a better relationship causes better adjustment.

Is relationship quality at Time 1 related to adjustment a year later? This question was important because we wanted to know whether the mother–child relationship early on in the divorce process might have far-reaching meaning for adjustment. As had been true within Time 1 and within Time 2, we found that mothers with higher self-reported mother–child relationship scores at Time 1 rated their children as having fewer behavior problems at Time 2, as did the children's teachers (see Appendix Table 7.5). Interestingly, what had appeared a high-quality observed relationship at Time 1 was now related to more behavior problems, as reported by mothers. Further, mothers' own psychological adjustment at Time 2 was significantly related to Time 1 (though, as shown above, not Time 2) mother–child relationship scores. That is, whether she felt good at Time 2 was related to how her relationship with her child had been a year earlier. One possible view of these results is that a mother's view of her child and of child rearing at a peak time of distress should be seen as an integral and far-reaching part of her psychological make-up.

MOTHERS' AND CHILDREN'S FAMILY LIVES AND RELATIONSHIP QUALITY

Having shown that both mothers' and children's adjustment were related to their relationship, we wanted to know more about what made a good relationship more likely. We looked first to several factors closely related to the mothers' and children's lives. Family systems-oriented clinical theories (e.g., Bowen, 1978; Minuchin, 1974) led us to predict that mothers and children might be free to have a better relationship with each other if (1) each of them individually had a better relationship with the father, (2) the child were not caught in loyalty struggles between the parents, and (3) they each had good support outside the family. We expected that if each of these conditions was true, the mother–child relationship would be able to blossom optimally. Thus, our analyses revolved around the question, "Do the relationships mothers and children have with others in their lives have a bearing on the relationship they have with each other?"

Measurement of Aspects of Mothers' and Children's Lives

To examine our first prediction, we needed a measure of the quality of the relationship between the mother and father, and between the child and father. We used a combined score of conflict and closeness for each dyad. For the *conflict* part of the score, we used the measure of interpersonal conflict (described in more detail in Chapter 5) coded from the interviews of mothers and all participating children, this time assessing both father–child and mother—father conflicts. Scores ranged from "no overt conflict with no apparent tension in the relationship" to "constant overt conflict."

To measure *closeness* between the mother and father and between the father and child, we again turned to the interviews of mothers and all participating children, and coded their answers to our questions about how the parents (or fathers and children) were getting along after the separation. Scores ranged on a 3-point scale for relations that are "close" ("I guess we're very good friends, very good friends . . . we're both, you know, happy with the way the other person's life is going . . . he's a wonderful listener now . . . it's very important to both of us to maintain that relationship now."), "neutral" ("They aren't sad but they aren't really excited; about the same except they aren't fighting; it's better."), or "separate" ("I was going to say there's no relationship, but I can't say there's no relationship. When we do see one another, it's very kind of short, cut and dried. And usually the conversation is just regarding Jason. I would say very strained, not at all friendly.").[3]

To examine the second prediction, mothers' and children's interviews were also coded for indicators that the child was involved in a *loyalty strain* between the parents. For example, we coded instances in which parents asked the child direct questions about the social lives of the other, admonishing him/her not to tell that they have done so, or in which parents directly asked the child which parent he/she likes better. One child said she frequently felt caught between her parents: "Like, a lot of times if I do something for my father, my mother will say, 'Oh, why do you like him more?' or 'Why didn't you do it for me, too?' Like the time I was in the Berkshires with my grandparents I wrote a postcard to my father. . . . And she just got, she was very upset about that. She was just asking me why. I felt bad—I felt bad that I didn't think of her." It was expected that children caught in this kind of dilemma would have a difficult time having an optimal relationship with their mothers (and their fathers).

To examine the third prediction, we coded mothers' and children's involvement outside the family, figuring that activities with job, school, or friends might help minimize the stress of the separation. Mothers' *extrafamilial involvement* was captured in a score that combined their ratings of occupational satisfaction and their reports of the amount of adult companionship they encountered. The children's extrafamilial involvement score included children's self-reported levels of school performance, activities with friends, and activities with nonparental adults.

In short, we asked whether the quality of the mother–child relationship was related to these seven aspects of the mothers' and children's relational lives:

- Interpersonal conflict between mother and father
- Closeness between mother and father
- Interpersonal conflict between child and father
- Closeness between child and father
- Loyalty strain
- Mother extrafamilial involvement
- Child extrafamilial involvement

As we had done in the previous section, we asked whether relationship quality was related to these aspects of the pairs' lives within Time 1, within Time 2, and over time (see Figure 7.2).[4] As no significant results were found

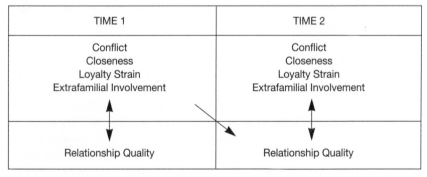

FIGURE 7.2. Analysis strategy: Links between relationship quality and family lives.

in the Time 1–Time 2 or within-Time 2 analyses, only the within-Time 1 results are discussed here (see also Appendix Table 7.6).

Within Time 1, the father–child conflict scores and the mothers' extrafamilial involvement were significantly related to the observational and self-report measures of relationship quality, respectively. Surprisingly, *higher* father–child conflict was related to *better* observed mother–child relationship scores. Although we had expected that lower conflict would leave children freer to have optimal relationships with their mothers, it seems that conflict with fathers marked a different kind of family dynamic instead. It may be that high conflict with fathers led to a kind of separation that was facilitative of—or perhaps a result of—a closer relationship with mothers. For example, high father–child conflict could be an indicator that the children felt "finished" with the father, as evidenced by their not wanting to visit him or by "hating him." This could be a temporary defense on their part, in which children are able to feel better about the separation; after all, they no longer have to live with the man with whom they had such conflict. Or it could free them to identify with the mothers' anger toward the fathers, thus being closer to the mothers. Alternately, the direction of causality could go the other way. Closeness to and identification with mothers could have resulted in higher father–child conflict, as the children took on their mothers' role in the relationship. In any case this seems to serve a temporary adaptive purpose rather than reflecting a permanent pattern, because the statistical link between father–child conflict and mother–child relationship was no longer significant by Time 2.

Yet another explanation of this finding is suggested by several families in which the mothers filed for divorce in reaction to destructive or disruptive behavior on the parts of the fathers. In one case, for example, the mother and children reported relief after the divorce, as they no longer had to deal daily with a "negative force," as the mother put it, of a "rigid, pressuring" husband. In helping the children manage the transition, this mother took a very active role in processing what was happening to the family, providing articulate expressions of her own and the children's reactions and trying consciously to create a supportive family life. The children saw their mother as resilient and protective and did not particularly want to "finish" their relationship with their father. Thus, children's conflict with the fathers may elicit highly proactive and supportive behavior from the mothers, resulting in high mother–child relationship quality.

Mothers with higher occupational satisfaction and social support had higher self-report relationship scores, more reflective of parental warmth and lack of distant and rigid control. The specificity of this relationship raises the question again of "reporter bias" as mothers were the sole contributors to both scores—do mothers who report being happy in one domain simply tend to report being happy in all domains? We doubt this possibility, however, because mothers' reports contributed to all of the other scores except child extrafamilial involvement, yet only this measure of extrafamilial involvement was significant. In this immediate postseparation time, the degree to which mothers' lives outside the family are satisfying is most predictive of the quality of their relationships with their children. In short, the finding may be interpreted as further evidence for the holistic nature of women's psychological experience—their relationships with their children, their parenting attitudes, their work, and their friends are all closely interwoven.

Perhaps even more interesting than these findings is that the quality of the mother–child relationship (which we know from the previous section continues to be linked to mothers' and children's adjustment) was no longer linked to relationships with the father or to social and job networks by Time 2. Apparently other dimensions had taken on increased importance in determining the nature of the mother–child relationship. We therefore turned to the broader context of the relationship to try to understand its nature.

BROADER FAMILY CONTEXTS AND RELATIONSHIP QUALITY

The mother–child relationship exists in a context, not in some psychological vacuum made up only of the individuals' identities. To broaden our examination of the mother–child relationship, we next undertook to assess how it might be related to the following:

- The family's place in the socioeconomic community
- The family's history of prior problems
- The adjustment of the other children

Measurement of Family Context Constructs

The family's *socioeconomic status (SES)* was measured using the Hollingshead and Redlich (1958) scale. Scores refer to the family's postseparation SES, based on mothers' occupation, derived separately at Time 1 and Time 2 based on information provided at those times.[5] The *family stress measure* was a count of the number of preseparation stresses the family had encountered, such as parental unemployment; legal, medical, or psychiatric difficulties of any family member; or substance abuse. The *sibling adjustment measure* was a combination of scores described above for the focus children, this time as a mean score of all variables for all nonfocus children in the family for whom we had data. Variables included their psychological adjustment (perceived competence, physical and psychological symptoms, and divorce-related affect), school performance, activities with friends, and activities with non-parental adults.

In this set of analyses, we were asking the question "Are family context measures related to the mother–child relationship quality?" within both times and over time[6] (see Figure 7.3). We found significant results only in the within-Time 2 analyses (see Appendix Table 7.7). Not surprisingly, there was a trend for families with less stressful histories to have better mother–child relationships. In addition, families in which the other siblings were doing well—psychologically, in school, with friends—tended to be those families in which the mothers and focus children had the best relationships. This is certainly consistent with a systemic view of the family as interconnected and reciprocally influential. In reviewing interviews with mothers who had high-quality relationships (according to our two scores) with their focus children, we found that these mothers articulated a clear sense of the distinctiveness of their children and their separate needs and, at the same time, offered an attentive and salient presence to all of their children. Expression of feelings, including anger and sadness, was highly valued. Families with lower-quality relationships between mothers and focus children and lower sibling adjustment tended not to have mothers who could tolerate and address the children's intense feelings. One such family, for example, was particularly unsettled and volatile, with the children collectively exposed to high parental conflict and the mother alternately being unavailable or present but enraged.

Finally, the SES results are interesting. The assessment of SES is based entirely on the status level of the mother's job; thus, it indexes her salary income and the occupational prestige of her job, but does not include any indication of income or resources the family may have available from the father. Mothers holding lower-SES jobs had child-rearing attitudes more reflective of a better relationship with their children (warmth, closeness, and a lack of emphasis on punishment). Athough this was surprising in the sense that fam-

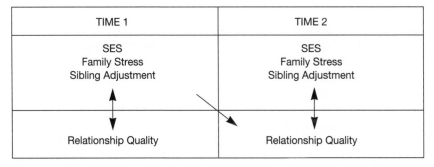

FIGURE 7.3. Analysis strategy: Links between relationship quality and broader family contexts.

ilies with fewer resources are often found to be more at risk for problems,[7] in our sample, work status and actual availability of money were at times inversely related to how important money seemed to be in influencing relationships. That is, in one family where the mother held a high-status job, the parents continued to fight angrily over money. The mother complained that the husband did not give her more money, that he "lied to the court" about how much money he had, and that he refused to pay a minor amount for an activity fee she felt her daughter needed, despite his having a good salary. In this family, the mother–child relationship was similarly quarrelsome and angry.

In contrast, in one family with low SES, the mother reported being quite unconcerned about money. Although she said that financially, "things [are] a lot tighter," her ex-husband was paying his (small) required child support regularly, they had a lifestyle that matched her means, and she was engaged, by Time 2, to another man who promised to watch over her financial needs. This mother's perception was that she had fewer money worries than before and that she spent more time with her children, about which they were "all excited." Thus, it seems that the SES groups may have viewed money differently, or perhaps they let it influence the kinds of relationships they had differently, despite any objective strain it presented to making ends meet.

In addition to these different attitudes about money among women with higher- and lower-status jobs, the differences in their attitudes about parenting may reflect broader differences in their ideas about how to help children cope with parental separation and divorce. It may be that women in higher-status jobs—which demand lots of independent coping—are more inclined to encourage children's independent coping efforts, a stance that might also be cooler and seem less sympathetic. In contrast, women in lower-status jobs may feel warmth and closeness are resources they can provide in an unlimited way to their children.

CONCLUSIONS

As we have shown, during the peak time of postseparation stress, the nature of the mother–child relationship was closely tied to the adjustment of both players. For both mothers and children, a better relationship (as tapped by our insider self-report measure) was related to better psychological adjustment—a construct that included self-reported descriptions of current psychological functioning, symptoms, and moods—but not to levels of physical illness. It was also related, for the children, to having fewer behavior problems, as rated by both teachers and mothers. The outsider observational view of the relationship was also related to the outsider (teacher) ratings of children's adjustment in a direction that suggests that children behave differently at home and at school. Thus, seen from inside and out, adjustment is embedded in relationships and should be understood in those terms. Taking care of the relationship is likely to facilitate better adjustment for both mothers and children, just as those who are feeling better are likely to get along better with each other.

After a year, only the children's behavior problems by the outsider's view continued to be significantly related to the nature of the relationship. The link to mothers' and children's self-reported psychological adjustment disappeared. Although at first glance it appears as if the nature of the relationship no longer mattered for mothers' adjustment, this conclusion would be premature. For both mothers and children, the link to self-reported feelings diminished while it remained for children's behavioral adjustment, so it may be that the relationship has overt consequences more than internal ones over time or with distance from the stressful separation. As we had no parallel, observable behavioral measure of mothers' adjustment, we cannot be sure of what impact the relationship may continue to have had for the mothers. Perhaps if we had had an outsider's view of the mothers—from friends, coworkers, or therapists, for example—we would have found at Time 2 that the mother–child relationship mattered for mothers' adjustment too.

In this light, it is interesting to speculate on the nature of the different adjustment measures we used. By Time 2, only children's behavior problems were related to the mother–child relationship. Perhaps this relatively objective report of adjustment is more robust and less likely to be altered by the moment-to-moment fluctuations in mood and attitude that might characterize the psychological adjustment measures. Even the pattern of good observed relationship quality being related to more teacher-rated behavior problems held through Time 2. Interestingly, those mothers who had been observed to have good relationships with their children at Time 1 rated their children as having more behavior problems at Time 2, coming into line with what the teachers had seen a year earlier. Further, though we have earlier considered mother ratings of behavior problems as an insider view (because mothers are inside the family), it might be useful here to note that they are both insider and outsider reports or in between the two, because mothers are also "outside" the child. By Time 2, when families may have reached some new level of adaptation, mothers may stand further apart from their children and, in this sense, give us an outsider's view of the child's adjustment.

It seems, then, that the rating of a more observable aspect of adjustment (i.e., behavior problems) continues over time to be related to the mother–child relationship. A different pattern emerges for the insider adjustment measures. At Time 1, the currents of stress and the mothers' concerns with safety, integrity, and survival may have been so strong as to keep insider relations between adjustment and mother–child relationship quite consistent. As these currents weakened with time, individual variations may have become the more important force, resulting in less striking links between

psychological adjustment and relationships. Those who would help understand women's and children's reactions to parental stress should be sure to
look broadly at different domains of adjustment.

More light is shed on this issue by other findings in this chapter. At Time
1, it was the aspects of the mothers' and children's direct relational lives (especially mothers' extrafamilial support and father–child conflict) that were
linked more strongly to the nature of the mother–child relationship than the
broader familial factors. By Time 2, this had reversed; socioeconomic factors,
family history, and sibling adjustment were significantly related to the relationship whereas the aspects of mothers' and children's relational lives were
not. The meaning of the mother–child relationship is thus critically reflective
of its time context. Put another way, distance from the separation seems to
play a role in affecting the meaning of the mother–child relationship. Further, it is clearly critical, if we are to understand individual adjustment, to
consider the broader contexts within which individuals live. Mothers' and
children's adjustment are linked to each other, apparently in the midst of
their relationships with the rest of their family and community.

It is important to note, too, that many of the things that affect relationship quality (and thus adjustment of both women and children) are not always under mothers' control, especially by themselves alone. Whether mothers were satisfied with their jobs, whether the children were in conflict with
or close to their fathers, the family's history of stresses, and the family's SES,
for example, are either difficult to change, dependent on outsiders for
change, or (in the case of family history of stresses) unchangeable. We hope
these findings can be useful in describing and understanding adjustment to
parental separation, but they should also release parents from feeling that
they can shoulder all the burden of their children's and their own adjustment.

Finally, it is important to note that the most striking and consistent
findings about the mother–child relationship were found in the first set of
analyses reported, those involving the mothers' and children's adjustment,
both within and across time. Children's behavior problems were related to
both self-reported and observed measures of mother–child relationship quality at both times (although mothers and teachers differed in their descriptions of children with better observed relationship quality, suggesting that
children behave differently in different settings). Further, mothers' Time 1
self-reported relationship quality was related to their own psychological adjustment at both times and to children's psychological adjustment at Time 1.
For both mothers and children, there appears to be some kind of unity between one's adjustment and one's view of one's mother–child relationship.
Personality has traditionally been examined in terms of individual-level constructs such as extraversion, conscientiousness, or agreeableness. Our data
support the suggestion that a relational element should be added to this con-

struction: women's and children's (and probably men's) selves are importantly, if partially, described by the nature of their close relationships (Chodorow,
1978; Gilligan, 1982; Lykes, 1985; Markus & Oyserman, 1989; Miller, 1986).
Just as it is important to family members' sense of self that they are, or aren't,
extraverted, conscientious, or agreeable, it may be critical that they have, or
don't have, effective, supportive, rewarding relationships with those people
who are important in their lives.

NOTES

1. See Copeland (1984) for a fuller explanation of the coding of these tapes. The summary score reported here was an aggregate of the mother interaction–child interaction,
child interaction–mother interaction, mother interaction–child no interaction, and
child interaction–mother no interaction codes. See Copeland (1984, 1985a, 1985b,
1990) for results of other analyses involving these interaction codes.

2. We performed six multiple regression analyses for each time period, with observed and
mother-reported relationship quality as the independent variables and each of the four
child and two mother adjustment measures as the dependent variables. Results are
shown in Appendix Tables 7.3, 7.4, and 7.5.

3. Interview transcripts were coded without knowledge of the coding of other variables.
Coding definitions and judgments were discussed for closeness and for loyalty strains,
until raters attained interrater reliability above .85; random spot checks of coding were
performed to ensure that reliability was maintained at or above this level.

4. We performed two multiple regression analyses for each time period, with the seven indicators of conflict, closeness, loyalty strain, and extrafamilial involvement as the independent variables and each of the two relationship quality measures as the dependent
variables. As no significant results were found in the Time 1–Time 2 or within-Time 2
analyses, only the within-Time 1 results are presented in Appendix Table 7.6.

5. This measure of SES based on mothers' occupation was significantly correlated with
mothers' educational level, $r(89) = .64$, $p < .001$; to fathers' occupational status measured on the same scale, $r(86) = .27$, $p < .05$; and to the family's available financial resources, $r(73) = .27$, $p < .05$.

6. We performed two multiple regression analyses for each time period, with SES, family
stress, and sibling adjustment as the independent variables and each of the two relationship quality measures as the dependent variables. As no significant results were
found in the within-Time 1 or Time 1–Time 2 analyses, only the within-Time 2 results
are presented in Appendix Table 7.7.

7. Indeed, in our sample, actual financial resources were negatively related to number of
teacher-rated behavior problems, $r(53) = -.31$, $p < .05$, and a coded score of "objective
financial deprivation" was positively correlated with mother-rated behavior problems,
$r(103) = .36$, $p < .001$, and mothers' illness, $r(88) = .26$, $p < .05$. When asked to compare
whether they or their ex-husbands were more financially deprived, mothers' reports of

"higher subjective deprivation" (relative to their husbands') were also related to child and mother adjustment, to mother-rated behavior problems, $r(103) = .32$, $p < .001$; mothers' psychological adjustment, $r(88) = -.24$, $p < .05$; and mothers' illness, $r(88) = .23$, $p < .05$. Thus, financial problems were related to more adjustment problems, but the findings reported in this section suggest that families in different SES groups may translate money concerns into relationship patterns differently.

CHAPTER 8

When the Conflict Continues

IMPLICATIONS OF PARENTAL CONFLICT IN THE POSTSEPARATION FAMILY

In Chapter 7, we examined the implications of the *mother–child dyad's functioning* for the adjustment of mothers and children. Here we will explore the implications of the *parental dyad's functioning* for family members' adjustment. This is, in a way, an odd topic because in theory the mother and father are *not* a dyad in the family any more. However, one of the distinguishing features of parental divorce, when compared with divorces of couples without children, is the need created by both parents' relationships to the same children for the parents to maintain some kind of relationship with each other. In Chapter 3 we saw that some parents found this difficult and painful, while others found it fairly easy. In Chapter 4 we saw that children were quite aware of their parents' postseparation relationship. And in Chapters 5 and 6, we discussed parental conflict as one of several factors related to adjustment problems for parents and children. We have, then, considerable reason to believe that the postseparation parental dyad's functioning—particularly conflict in that relationship—is an important factor in family members' adjustment. In this chapter, we change our lens and focus on the broad pattern of relationships between parental conflict and children's adjustment. In Chapter 9, we will examine patterns of conflict and parenting more thoroughly among the 22 couples in which both the mother and the father participated in our study over time.

This chapter was drafted by Nicole B. Barenbaum.

While it seems obvious that most divorcing spouses are in conflict with each other, we have also seen that there are differences among divorcing couples (as there are among couples who do not divorce) with respect to the level of conflict in the relationship and the ways they handle the conflict. Some couples argue constantly (as one mother put it, the "screaming and yelling has been going on half our married life"). Some have physical confrontations, while still others grow apart, losing emotional contact without a great deal of arguing or physical aggression (e.g., one husband in our study was surprised when his wife raised the subject of separation because there had been no overt conflict between them, but his wife felt that the lack of emotional contact in their relationship was intolerable). It seemed important, then, to look more closely at the effects of different types of conflict to discover whether some types were particularly harmful. For example, violent confrontations between parents might have especially negative effects on children's adjustment, whereas legal battles over division of property (if overt conflict between the parents is limited) might not. Conflict (like parents' and children's adjustment) is multifaceted and parents may be involved in many different types of conflict as they go through the process of divorce during the postseparation period.

We assessed several types of conflict from different sources, in order to get as complete a picture as possible (see Table 8.1). Of particular interest was the level of *overt conflict and violence* between parents. This type of conflict, if children are aware of it, might be especially upsetting to them; on the other hand, if the separation puts an end to violent confrontations, children might be relieved during the postseparation period. We asked parents to complete a

TABLE 8.1. Measures of Parental Conflict

Overt conflict

- CTS—questionnaire completed by couple for last year of marriage; two subscales:
  Verbal reasoning
  Violence
- Couple violent—coded from interviews
- Restraining or vacating orders

Legal conflict

- Number of legal motions—coded from court records
  Child-related motions (custody, visitation, or support)
  Restraining or vacating orders
- Divorce heard in court?

Interpersonal conflict

- Composite of custodial mother's and children's views of parental relationship standard questionnaire describing specific ways they had handled disagreements with one another during the last year of the marriage (Conflict Tactics Scale [CTS]; Straus, 1974, 1979). One scale from this measure assessed violence (e.g., "pushed, grabbed, or shoved him/her"), while another assessed verbal reasoning (e.g., "tried to discuss the issue calmly"). We also assessed violence from the interviews, in which parents sometimes described violent episodes or patterns, in the context of describing the history of their relationship and how they handled conflict. As a third indicator of overt conflict, we looked at the number of legal motions for restraining and vacating orders the couple had filed in court. We saw these as representing parents' efforts to prevent physical confrontations with their spouses, as well as their inability to resolve a conflict about which parent should leave the marital home.

In addition, we assessed the overall level of *legal conflict* between the parents from court records dating from the time of filing for the divorce until Time 2. Legal actions might be used by some parents as a vehicle for the expression of conflict—one that might be less obvious to children. On the other hand, legal actions might be related to overt conflict (as in the case of motions for restraining and vacating orders), and they might involve the children directly (as in the case of custody disputes). For these reasons, we assessed the number of legal motions in these categories separately as well.

We also recorded whether the divorce had been heard in court by the time of the follow-up interview. Although the divorce was not considered final until at least 6 months after the date of the court hearing, the hearing generally marked the settlement of legal issues such as disposition of property, custody, and visitation. Many of our participants experienced the hearing as an important transition and considered the waiting period to be just a formality. Therefore, we were interested in comparing families who had passed this transition point with those who had not.

Finally, as is described in Chapters 5 and 6, we assessed family members' perceptions of the level of *interpersonal conflict* between the parents.[1] Even in the absence of overt conflict, it may be obvious that parents are not getting along; as one mother said, "If he was downstairs watching TV, I'd go to bed. If he went to bed, I'd go downstairs and watch TV." Thus, not only family members who witness verbal and physical confrontations, but also those who are aware of tension and distance between the parents, may report high levels of interpersonal conflict. Children living in a family in which members perceive a high level of parental conflict might be expected to suffer some negative effects as long as that conflict continues. On the other hand, children whose parents' relationship after separation is extremely amicable might become confused about why a separation is necessary.

In this chapter we will not examine the effects of conflict directly involving the children, that is, instances in which children become allied with one parent against the other (loyalty strains). Although loyalty strains represent an important aspect of conflict that clearly affects children's postseparation adjustment (as we saw in Chapter 6), we will concentrate here on the conflict in the divorcing parent dyad and discuss the effects of loyalty strains in Chapter 10, which focuses on family (rather than dyadic) interaction patterns.

First we will explore *relationships among different types of conflict.* Next, we will ask several important questions concerning the *consequences of parental conflict for children.* Studies of both "intact" and divorced families have found that parental conflict has negative effects on children (see, e.g., Emery, 1982, and Fincham, Grych, & Osborne, 1994, for reviews); in fact, parental conflict has sometimes been found to have more negative consequences than divorce itself (i.e., children in "intact" families with high levels of parental conflict show poorer adjustment than those in divorced families with low levels of parental conflict). Also, custody battles between divorcing parents have been found to affect children negatively. But do different types of conflict have different consequences for children's adjustment during the postseparation period? Does conflict have both short- and longer-term consequences for children? Does conflict have the same effects for boys and girls, and for children of different ages? Are children whose parents settle their divorces relatively quickly less affected by parental conflict than those whose parents do not?

Conflict may also affect children indirectly if it affects their parents' adjustment, as children's well-being following the separation is at least somewhat related to the adjustment of their custodial parents. Therefore, we will also explore the *impact of different types of conflict on parents' adjustment.*

Finally, we will explore *characteristics of parents, families, and couples associated with different types of conflict.* For example, parents with particular motive patterns might be expected to use more aggressive conflict tactics than others, or families with financial problems might have more legal conflict regarding support payments than others. Understanding these kinds of relationships might help us to identify families at risk for developing high levels of conflict or destructive conflict tactics.

ARE DIFFERENT TYPES OF CONFLICT RELATED TO EACH OTHER?

For mothers, there were several significant relationships among indicators of overt conflict (see Appendix Table 8.1). Mothers who reported violence in their interviews also reported higher violence on the CTS and had more legal conflict at Time 1 (and more motions for vacating and restraining orders at both times[2]). However, CTS scores were unrelated to legal conflict. Among our smaller sample of fathers, there were fewer relationships among different types of conflict (see Appendix Table 8.2). CTS violence scores and family reports of interpersonal conflict at Time 1 were related to higher levels of legal conflict at Time 2.

About two-thirds of the families who returned at Time 2 to participate in our study had settled their divorces in court by this time. Both mothers and fathers whose divorces had been settled by Time 2 had lower levels of some types of conflict than those whose divorces remained unsettled.[3] Mothers who had settled the divorce had higher CTS verbal reasoning scores, lower levels of interpersonal conflict, and fewer legal motions related to children (those regarding custody, support, or visitation) by Time 2,[4] than those whose divorces had not been settled. Among mothers, then, it is possible that lower levels of conflict facilitated the divorce settlement, or that the settlement helped to reduce conflict, or both.

Fathers whose family members reported lower levels of interpersonal conflict at both times were more likely to have reached a divorce settlement by Time 2 than those with higher levels of interpersonal conflict. For fathers, it appears that lower levels of interpersonal conflict at Time 1 facilitated settling the divorce, which in turn may have helped to maintain lower levels of interpersonal conflict at Time 2.

HOW DOES PARENTAL CONFLICT RELATE TO CHILDREN'S ADJUSTMENT?

For children of custodial mothers, we looked at relationships between the various indicators of conflict and adjustment (see Table 8.2 and Appendix Table 8.3). It is clear from these results that parental conflict involving physi-

TABLE 8.2. Relationships between Parental Conflict and Children's Adjustment, All Children ($n = 120$)

Self-report	Mother report		Teacher report
Psychological adjustment	Illness	Behavior problems	Behavior problems
		Time 1	
No relationships	No relationships		Husband violent
		Total legal motions	
		Vacating/restraining motions	
		Time 2	
Interpersonal conflict Time 2 (negative)	No relationships	Total legal motions Time 1	CTS violence
		Vacating/restraining motions Time 1	Interpersonal conflict Time 2

Note. Negative relationships with adjustment indicate that conflict is associated with poor psychological adjustment (self-report).

cal aggression was related to behavior problems for children, both at Time 1 and over time.

Time 1

At Time 1, children's behavior problems at home (according to their mothers) and at school (according to their teachers) were related to several indicators of overt conflict between parents. Relationships between children's behavior problems and parents' legal conflict were largely due to relationships between behavior problems and the number of motions for vacating and restraining orders, an indicator of actual or feared aggression. Children's psychological adjustment was generally unrelated to parental conflict at Time 1, possibly because children were more focused on the immediate changes in their daily lives at this time, or because some felt relieved by the separation, hoping it would put an end to the fighting. Unlike the various indicators of overt conflict, interpersonal conflict between parents, as reported by family members at Time 1, was unrelated to children's adjustment.

Over-Time Effects

Overt conflict between parents before the separation also had long-term effects on children's behavior problems at home and at school at Time 2.

Time 2

In contrast to the absence of relationships between interpersonal conflict and children's adjustment within Time 1 or over time, we found relationships between parents' interpersonal conflict at Time 2 and their children's poor psychological adjustment and behavior problems at school. Perhaps this type of parental conflict was unrelated to children's adjustment until later because the children were preoccupied with the changes in their daily routines early in the postseparation period and turned their attention to more subtle aspects of their parents' relationship only after they had begun to adjust to these changes. Alternatively, children may have become habituated to this type of conflict between their parents during the period before the separation so that it did not have much of an impact immediately after the separation. A year later, persistent interpersonal conflict may have had more of an impact, because children had become less habituated to it (e.g., if they observed it less frequently), because they were themselves drawn into it more, or because they were disappointed in their expectation that the separation would help to decrease the level of conflict between their parents. Effects of interpersonal conflict, which may have included less aggressive forms of conflict, seem to have been more internalized, resulting in psychological problems as well as behavior problems.

In sum, parents' overt conflict at Time 1 had both short- and longer-term effects on their children's behavior problems. Interpersonal conflict, which may have been less overt, was unrelated to children's adjustment until Time 2, when it was related to behavior problems and to poor psychological adjustment.

DID CHILDREN DIFFER BY AGE AND GENDER IN THEIR RESPONSES TO PARENTAL CONFLICT?

When we looked at relationships between parental conflict and adjustment for different groups of children, some interesting patterns emerged. The adjustment of older children (ages 9–12) was less related to parental conflict than that of younger children (ages 6–8), and boys and girls responded in different ways to different types of conflict. Boys' adjustment was related to parents' legal conflict and their specific conflict tactics (see Table 8.3 and Appendix Table 8.4).

Younger Boys

At Time 1, younger boys had more behavior problems at school if their parents had made many legal motions for vacating or restraining orders or many motions related to custody; custody motions were also related to poor self-reported psychological adjustment. Over time, custody motions were related to behavior problems at home; this relationship also appeared within Time 2. For younger boys, then, custody battles appeared to be particularly upsetting. Younger boys also showed longer-term positive effects of earlier conflict tactics; that is, those boys whose parents had used more verbal reasoning during the last year of the marriage had fewer behavior problems at school at Time 2 than those whose parents had used less verbal reasoning.

Older Boys

Older boys' adjustment was also related to legal conflict and to specific conflict tactics, but in different ways than that of younger boys. At Time 1, older boys whose parents had made many motions for custody had *fewer* behavior

TABLE 8.3. Relationships between Parental Conflict and Adjustment, Boys

Self-report		Mother report				Teacher report	
Psychological adjustment		Illness		Behavior problems		Behavior problems	
Time 1	Time 2	Time 1	Time 2	Time 1	Time 2	Time 1	Time 2
Younger boys (ages 6–8) (n = 29)							
Custody motions Time 1 (negative)	No relationships	No relationships	No relationships	No relationships	Total legal motions Times 1, 2 Custody motions Times 1, 2	Vacating/ restraining motions Time 1 Custody motions Time 1	CTS verbal reasoning Time 1 (negative)
Older boys (ages 9–12) (n = 33)							
No relationships	No relationships	Custody motions Time 1 (negative)	No relationships	No relationships	No relationships	Total legal motions Time 1 (negative) Custody motions Time 1 (negative)	CTS violence Time 1

Note. Negative relationships with adjustment indicate that conflict is associated with poor psychological adjustment (self-report). Negative relationships with illness and behavior problems indicate that reasoning is related to better adjustment.

problems at school and *fewer* illnesses than those whose parents had not. Older and younger boys, then, reacted differently to parents' legal battles over custody. (We have seen in Chapter 3 that these battles were more common in families where there were boys than in families without boys.) The younger boys may have felt threatened by these battles, feeling that they were not ready to leave their mothers, while the older boys may have been more interested in going to live with their fathers. Other research has found that older boys are more likely to live with their fathers than are younger ones (see Emery, 1988).

Older boys whose parents had used violence as a conflict tactic during the last year of marriage showed more behavior problems at school at Time 2 than those whose parents had not. Older boys, then, showed effects of early overt conflict later than younger boys, and they did not show the same positive effect of verbal reasoning.

Girls' adjustment was related to parental conflict at both times, and in different ways than that of boys. For girls, all types of parental conflict (including overt conflict tactics, legal conflict, and family members' assessments of interpersonal conflict) were related to illness and psychological adjustment, but not to behavior problems. Younger girls' adjustment was related to parental conflict in more ways than that of older girls (see Table 8.4).

Younger Girls

At Time 1, younger girls had fewer illnesses if their parents had high verbal reasoning scores on the CTS, and more illnesses if interpersonal conflict between their parents was high. Both interpersonal conflict and violent conflict between parents had over-time effects on younger girls' illness at Time 2. In contrast, verbal reasoning had a positive over-time effect on younger girls' psychological adjustment.

Within Time 2, legal conflict was related to younger girls' illness, and interpersonal conflict was related to poor psychological adjustment. Also, those whose parents had settled their divorces by Time 2 showed better psychological adjustment than those whose parents were still not divorced.[5]

Older Girls

Older girls showed a similar pattern of relationships between parental conflict and adjustment to that of younger girls, although the relationships were fewer. At Time 1, older girls had more illnesses if legal conflict was high or if

TABLE 8.4. Relationships between Parental Conflict and Adjustment, Girls

	Self-report		Mother report		Mother report, teacher report	
	Psychological adjustment		Illness		Behavior problems	
	Time 1	Time 2	Time 1	Time 2	Time 1	Time 2
Younger girls (ages 6–8) (n = 30)						
	No relationships	CTS verbal reasoning Time 1 (negative)	CTS verbal reasoning Time 1 (negative)	Vacationing/restraining motions Time 1	No relationships	No relationships
		Interpersonal conflict Time 2 (negative)	Interpersonal conflict Time 1	Interpersonal conflict Time 1		
			Husband violent Time 1	Husband violent Time 1		
			Total legal motions Time 1	Total legal motions Time 2		
Older girls (ages 9–12) (n = 28)						
	No relationships	Interpersonal conflict Time 2 (negative)	Total legal motions Time 1	No relationships	No relationships	No relationships
			Husband violent Time 1			

Note. Negative relationships with adjustment indicate that conflict is associated with poor psychological adjustment (self-report). Negative relationships with illness indicate that reasoning is related to better adjustment.

their mothers had reported physical violence by their fathers, but adjustment at Time 2 was unrelated to conflict at Time 1. At Time 2, family reports of high interpersonal conflict were related to poorer psychological adjustment for older girls, as they were for younger girls.

The clear differences we found between boys' and girls' adjustment problems in relationship to parental conflict seem consistent with the differences in overall level of illness and behavior problems at school reported in Chapter 6. Parental conflict was generally related to externalizing (behavior problems) among boys and to internalizing (illness at both times, psychological distress at Time 2) among girls; important exceptions were custody motions at Time 1, which were related to younger boys' psychological distress and to older boys' physical health. These differences may reflect differences in specific responses to parental conflict. However, it is also possible that they reflect differences in willingness to report various types of problems when parental conflict is high. For example, girls may be more willing than boys to report psychological distress and physical symptoms; mothers and teachers may be more willing to report (or more likely to notice) behavior problems for boys than for girls. Also, in our sample of children in the custody of their mothers, girls may have identified more than boys with the custodial parent (and mothers may have had more of a tendency to perceive boys' behavior negatively). Unfortunately, our sample of children in the custody of their fathers was too small to permit comparable analyses.

Girls were affected not only by conflict tactics and legal conflict (as boys were), but also by interpersonal conflict, which may have been less overt. This pattern is consistent with research suggesting that girls are more responsive to family relationships, perhaps because they are more sheltered and socialized to be oriented toward family life than are boys (see, e.g., Block, 1984). Younger boys and girls seemed to be more affected by parental conflict than older ones, most likely because older children were less oriented toward the family and more involved with peers and activities away from home. Also, younger children, unlike older ones, showed positive effects of parents' verbal reasoning before the separation, again suggesting that they had been more oriented toward the family than were older children.

In sum, both younger and older boys had more behavior problems if their parents had high levels of overt conflict. In contrast, younger sons of parents who had engaged in custody disputes showed poorer psychological adjustment, while older sons showed fewer illnesses. Daughters in both age groups were affected by parents' interpersonal conflict, as well as by overt conflict and by legal disputes. Parental conflict was related to girls' illness and poor psychological adjustment, rather than to behavior problems, as it was for boys. Younger children of both sexes were more affected by parental conflict than were older children, especially by Time 2.

WHAT WERE CHILDREN'S RESPONSES TO CONFLICT AFTER THE DIVORCE WAS SETTLED?

It seemed reasonable to expect that children whose parents had settled the divorce would be less affected by parental conflict than those who were still in transition. Indeed, we found that the adjustment of children whose parents had settled the divorce was unrelated to parental conflict; the only exception was that children of parents who had high verbal reasoning scores on the CTS showed better psychological adjustment at Time 2 than those whose parents had used less verbal reasoning (see Table 8.5 and Appendix Table 8.5). In contrast, children whose parents had not settled the divorce by Time 2 showed long-term effects of earlier parental conflict, *and* their adjustment was *also* related to concurrent parental conflict at Time 2. These children were particularly affected by parental conflict involving violence or threats of violence, showing poorer psychological adjustment and more behavior problems at home and at school if overt conflict was high. It is important to note that parents in families where the divorce was settled did not have higher or lower levels of conflict overall; it was the relationship between parental conflict and children's adjustment that differed in these two kinds of families.

The divorce settlement, then, did appear to mark a transition for children—a lowering of children's vulnerability to conflict between their parents.

TABLE 8.5. Relationships between Parental Conflict and Children's Time 2 Adjustment, by Divorce Status

Self-report	Mother report		Teacher report
Psychological adjustment	Illness	Behavior problems	Behavior problems
Divorce settled by Time 2 (n = 51)			
CTS verbal reasoning	No relationships	No relationships	No relationships
Divorce unsettled by Time 2 (n = 46)			
Vacating/restraining motions Times 1, 2 (negative)	No relationships	Total legal motions Times 1, 2	CTS violence
		Vacating/restraining motions Times 1, 2	

Note. Negative relationships with adjustment indicate that conflict is associated with poor psychological adjustment (self-report).

It is important to remember that, in families in which the divorce remained unsettled at Time 2, interpersonal conflict reported by family members was higher than in those in which the divorce had been settled. Children in these families, then, may have been more sensitive to other types of conflict because of the context of higher conflict. Also, parents in these families had higher levels of legal conflict concerning children (i.e., motions regarding custody, support, and visitation)[6]; these children may have been directly affected by parental conflict in a way that other children were not, making them more responsive to aggressive conflict.

WAS PARENTAL CONFLICT RELATED TO PARENTS' ADJUSTMENT?

Children's well-being after separation was related to their mothers' adjustment. Therefore, parental conflict could affect children both directly and indirectly through their mothers' adjustment, if mothers were also adversely affected by conflict. In fact, mothers' adjustment was related to different types of parental conflict than was children's (see Table 8.6 and Appendix Table 8.6). We were equally interested in the connections between fathers' adjustment and parental conflict.

Mothers

At Time 1, mothers with high CTS verbal reasoning scores for the couple had better psychological adjustment and less illness than those who report-

TABLE 8.6. Relationships between Parental Conflict and Adjustment, Mothers ($n = 120$)

Psychological adjustment		Illness	
Time 1	Time 2	Time 1	Time 2
Child-related legal motions[a] (negative)	No relationships	CTS verbal reasoning (negative)	Interpersonal conflict Time 1
CTS verbal reasoning			Child-related legal motions Time 2

Note. Negative relationships with adjustment indicate that conflict is associated with poor psychological adjustment (self-report). Negative relationships with illness indicate that reasoning is related to better adjustment.

[a]Motions concerning support, custody, and/or visitation.

ed less verbal reasoning. However, mothers' adjustment, unlike that of their children, was unrelated to any indicators of overt conflict or violence. Although we might expect aggressive conflict to have negative consequences for mothers, it is possible that some mothers who had experienced abusive relationships were relieved to escape them and empowered by their decision to do so. Mothers reported poor psychological adjustment at Time 1 if there had been a large number of legal motions related to the children (i.e., motions regarding custody, support, or visitation). Custody motions alone were not related to mothers' adjustment, so this relationship was due largely to the relationship with the number of motions concerning support and/or visitation.

Although interpersonal conflict at Time 1 was unrelated to mothers' adjustment at that time, it appeared to have a long-term effect on their illness at Time 2. Possibly, the added strain of conflict with their ex-husbands while they were trying to establish the postseparation household eventually contributed to health problems for these mothers.

At Time 2, mothers reported more illness if legal conflict related to the children was high. As at Time 1, this relationship between legal conflict and mothers' adjustment was due largely to the relationship with the number of motions concerning support and/or visitation. It seems clear, then, that legal conflict over issues concerning the children, which may have interfered with mothers' efforts to care for the postseparation family, had negative consequences for them. Interpersonal conflict at Time 2 was unrelated to mothers' adjustment, and there were no differences in adjustment between mothers whose divorces had been settled and those whose divorces remained unsettled.[7]

Fathers

There were no relationships between fathers' adjustment and any type of conflict at either time. However, at Time 2, fathers whose divorces had been settled had fewer illnesses than those whose divorces had not yet been settled.[8] We cannot tell from this analysis whether illness was a result or a cause of the lack of resolution of the divorce.

In sum, mothers' adjustment was affected most by legal conflict threatening support or visitation. However, both parents' adjustment was generally less closely tied to other forms of interparental conflict—particularly violent or aggressive conflict—than was children's. This may be due to the normative nature of conflict in the context of divorce, or to parents' lessened investment in their relationship with one another. In any case, one benefit of this relative imperviousness is that parental conflict does not routinely put children in *double* jeopardy, through effects on their parents as well as direct effects on them. On the other hand, legal conflict about the children does seem to do just that.

DID THE DIVORCE SETTLEMENT AFFECT THE RELATIONSHIP BETWEEN PARENTAL CONFLICT AND PARENTS' ADJUSTMENT?

Mothers whose divorces had not been settled by Time 2 were more responsive to legal conflict related to children (i.e., motions regarding custody, support, or visitation); those with more legal motions related to children had poorer psychological adjustment and more illness than those with fewer such motions (see Table 8.7 and Appendix Table 8.6). Legal conflict involving the children, then, was particularly distressing to these mothers and may have been impeding the progress of the divorce settlement, as well as their efforts to establish routines and to provide for their families. (It is important to remember that families in which the divorce had not been settled by Time 2 generally had higher levels of legal conflict related to children than those in which the divorce had been settled.)

Interestingly, for mothers whose divorces *had* been settled by Time 2, psychological adjustment was poorer if interpersonal conflict reported by family members at Time 2 was high than if it was not. These mothers may have expected that the divorce settlement would decrease the level of parental conflict and may have been particularly discouraged if it did not. There were no other relationships between parental conflict and adjustment for this group.

TABLE 8.7. Relationships between Parental Conflict and Mothers' Time 2 Adjustment, by Divorce Status

Psychological adjustment	Illness
Divorce settled by Time 2 ($n = 51$)	
Interpersonal conflict Time 2 (negative)	No relationships
Divorce unsettled by Time 2 ($n = 46$)	
Child-related legal motions[a] Times 1, 2 (negative)	Child-related legal motions Time 2

Note. Negative relationships with adjustment indicate that conflict is associated with poor psychological adjustment (self-report).
[a]Motions concerning support, custody, and/or visitation.

WHICH PARENTS, FAMILIES, AND COUPLES HAD MORE PARENTAL CONFLICT?

Given that the different types of conflict and conflict tactics were related to children's and mothers' adjustment, we asked whether some parents (or parents in some situations) were more likely than others to experience these different types of conflict (see Tables 8.8 and 8.9, and Appendix Table 8.7).

TABLE 8.8. Predictors of Conflict, Mothers ($n = 120$)

	CTS	Violence index	Legal		Family
Level of predictor variable	Reasoning	Violence/ threats of violence[a]	Total motions	Child-related motions[b]	Interpersonal conflict
Individual		Spouse blame	Spouse blame		
		Low self-blame			
	High power motive/low responsibility (negative)	High power motive/low responsibility	High power motive/low responsibility		High power motive/low responsibility
				Trouble with necessities	
Family		Parental substance abuse and/or violence			
Couple		Previous marriage			
	Years married without children	Fewer years married without children			
	Mother changed status				Father's job status not higher than mother's
	Coparenting	Poor coparenting	Poor coparenting		Poor coparenting
		No mutual plans	No mutual plans		

[a]CTS violence, mother reports of father violence, legal motions for vacating/restraining orders.
[b]Motions concerning support, custody, and/or visitation.

TABLE 8.9. Predictors of Conflict, Fathers ($n = 34$)

Level of predictor variable	CTS Reasoning	Violence index Violence/ threats of violence[a]	Legal Total motions	Child-related motions[b]	Family Interpersonal conflict
Individual					Spouse blame
	High power motive/high responsibility (negative score)	High power motive/low responsibility			
Family		Parental substance abuse and/or violence			
Couple		Father's job status not higher than mother's	Father's job status not higher than mother's		
		Mother changed status	Mother changed status		
		Poor coparenting	Poor coparenting	Poor coparenting	Poor coparenting
		No mutual plans		No mutual plans	No mutual plans

[a]CTS violence, legal motions for vacating/restraining orders.
[b]Motions concerning support, custody, and/or visitation.

Individual Characteristics

We examined patterns of attributing blame for the divorce, because blaming one another might exacerbate hostility between divorcing spouses.[9] Mothers who attributed blame to their husbands (i.e., who mentioned many reasons for the divorce that blamed their husbands) reported more aggressive conflict tactics than those who attributed less blame to their husbands. They also had higher levels of legal conflict, especially legal conflict related to violence or threats of violence. For mothers, blaming their ex-spouses seemed to be not so much a predictor of conflict as a reflection of violence in the marriage. However, it is interesting that women who had experienced violence did *not* generally blame themselves, as is sometimes suggested. Self-blame (the number of reasons for which mothers blamed themselves) was largely unrelated to the different types of conflict, but mothers who had more motions for vacating and restraining orders at Time 1 blamed themselves *less* than other mothers. Perhaps some of the women in our sample who had decided not to stay with violent husbands blamed their husbands instead of themselves. Blaming the spouse may have helped them make the decision to divorce and may have protected them against internalizing in response to aggressive conflict or abuse; as discussed above, aggressive conflict was unrelated to mothers' adjustment.

Among fathers, in contrast, those who mentioned more reasons for the divorce blaming their wives had higher levels of interpersonal conflict according to family members at Time 1 than those who blamed their wives less, but there were no relationships between blaming the spouse and aggressive conflict. For fathers, blaming the spouse may have been a result of high levels of interpersonal conflict, or it may have contributed to that conflict.

Power motivation and responsibility were important predictors of conflict for mothers.[10] Earlier research has shown that individuals high in both power motivation and responsibility use socially acceptable strategies to influence others, while those high in power motivation but low in responsiblity use more impulsive and aggressive strategies (Winter & Barenbaum, 1985). Therefore, we expected that parents high in power motivation but low in responsibility would use more aggressive conflict tactics and have higher levels of conflict than those high in both power motivation and responsibility. We found that mothers who were high in power motivation and low in responsibility reported less verbal reasoning and more violence than mothers without this motive pattern. They also had more legal conflict and higher levels of interpersonal conflict at Time 1 than other mothers.[11] Thus, at Time 1 mothers with this motive pattern had higher levels of conflict of all types than other mothers. These mothers seem to have had a tendency to become involved not only in legal conflict, but also in hostile interchanges with their husbands, which then escalated into physical aggression. However, at Time 2 there were no differences between mothers with and those without this motive pattern.

Among fathers, those who were high in power motivation and low in responsibility had more legal motions for vacating and restraining orders at Time 2 than fathers without this motive pattern.[12] Thus, among both fathers and mothers, those with high power motivation and low responsibility had been involved in legal and interpersonal conflict often involving violence or threats of violence. However, unexpectedly, fathers who had high power motivation and *high* responsibility had *lower* verbal reasoning scores for the couple on the CTS than those without this motive pattern. This relationship reflects a general tendency among fathers high in responsibility to use less verbal reasoning.[13] Although we had expected fathers high in responsibility to use verbal reasoning (a conflict tactic requiring self-control and concern for others), the results suggest that these fathers may have reacted to conflict by internalizing or inhibiting any hostile impulses, rather than by attempting to reason with their spouses.

Financial Situation

The family's early financial situation was generally unrelated to parental conflict at either time. But at Time 2, mothers who reported problems obtaining basic necessities (e.g., food, housing, transportation) came from couples that made more legal motions related to children (particularly regarding support and visitation) than those who were more financially secure. There were no relationships between fathers' reports of financial difficulty and any type of conflict.

Family Characteristics

Families in which at least one *child* had had problems, including physical or emotional problems, legal problems, or substance abuse, did not have higher levels of the types of parental conflict we examine in this chapter. However, familes in which either *parent* had a history of physical violence or of substance abuse had higher levels of overt conflict at both times than other families, as indicated by their CTS violence scores and by their legal motions for vacating and restraining orders.

Several other family characteristics were unrelated to any type of parental conflict for either mothers or fathers. These included the age and sex distribution of children in the family and the number of recent losses suffered by either parent. Among fathers, custodial arrangements were unrelated to any type of conflict.

Couple Characteristics

Among mothers, two aspects of the parents' earlier marital history were related to conflict. Mothers from couples in which either spouse had been married previously were more likely than others to mention physical violence on the part of their husbands.[14] Mothers who had been married longer before any children were born reported more verbal reasoning and less violence on the CTS than mothers who had had children earlier in their marriages.[15] Among fathers, the parents' earlier marital history was unrelated to any type of conflict.

Aspects of the spouses' relative SES were related to conflict for both mothers and fathers; generally, couples with less traditional marital roles had higher levels of conflict than those with traditional roles. We compared the SES of each participant's job with that of his/her spouse, assigning a code of 1 if the participant's job status was higher, 2 if the two were equal, and 3 if the spouse's job status was higher. For both mothers and fathers, conflict was generally greater if the mother's job status was higher than or equal to the father's than if the father's job status was higher. Similarly, fathers whose wives had been students or had changed jobs before the separation (perhaps reflecting their efforts to improve their status relative to that of their husbands) had more legal conflict than fathers whose wives had not attempted to change their status. These findings are consistent with earlier research showing that divorce is more likely when the ratio of wives' income relative to that of their husbands is greater (see Raschke, 1987, for a review).

Among our divorcing couples, then, women who earned as much as (or more than) their husbands may have been more willing to engage in conflict than those who did not. However, unlike the wives of fathers in our study, mothers who had been students or had changed jobs before the separation reported more verbal reasoning on the CTS than those who had not, but not higher levels of conflict than other mothers.

We expected that parents who were able to cooperate in matters concerning the children would have lower levels of conflict than those who were not. Coparenting relationships, coded from the parent interviews, were defined as "poor" if the parents disagreed about child-rearing issues or visitation and had difficulty resolving these disagreements, or as "good" if there was no evidence of conflict related to child-rearing issues or if parents mentioned explicitly that they cooperated on issues regarding the children.[16] For both mothers and fathers, better coparenting relationships at Time 1 were related to lower levels of violent and interpersonal conflict at Time 1 and to lower levels of legal conflict at Time 2. For mothers, better coparenting at Time 2 was related to less legal and interpersonal conflict. Of course, we cannot tell whether better coparenting contributed to lower levels of conflict or vice versa. Similarly, mothers and fathers who mentioned in their interviews that they had made mutual plans with their spouses before the separation (regarding custody and living arrangements) had lower levels of violence and less legal conflict at both times than those who had not.[17] Fathers who had made mutual plans also had lower levels of interpersonal conflict at Time 1 than those who had not. Clearly, then, parents who were able to communicate well enough to make decisions together regarding the separation itself and the children's welfare were able to minimize all three types of conflict.

In sum, a number of characteristics of individuals, families, and couples predicted parental conflict. Spouse blame was related to violent conflict among mothers and to interpersonal conflict among fathers. Mothers with high power motivation and low responsibility had more conflict of all types than other mothers, and fathers with this motive pattern were involved with more legal motions for vacating and restraining orders than other fathers. Among mothers, the number of years married before children were born was related to lower levels of aggressive conflict, and previous marriage of either spouse was related to higher levels of aggressive conflict. Among both mothers and fathers, couples with less traditional marital roles with respect to the relative SES of their jobs had more conflict than those with more traditional roles. Also among both mothers and fathers, good coparenting and mutual planning for the divorce were related to lower levels of all types of conflict.

CONCLUSIONS

It is clear from the results reported in this chapter that high levels of parental conflict did have negative consequences for children, although the consequences of parental conflict differed for different groups of children. Aggressive conflict early in the separation process was particularly problematic for children's adjustment. It may be that after their parents' separation, children are especially vulnerable to parental conflict, given their increased passive receptivity (described in Chapter 4). Ironically, parents may be unusually prone to expressing conflict directly because of *their* particularly proactive orientation at the same time (see Chapter 3).

Gender also mattered in children's responses to conflict, and in their parents'. Boys and girls of different ages responded differently to different types of conflict, in ways that echo the age and gender differences reported in Chapters 4 and 6. First, older children were less affected by parental conflict than younger children. Among boys, conflict was mostly related to behavior problems, but among girls it was related to illness and psychological adjustment. (The connection with illness for girls is mirrored in the results for mothers.) Finally, boys' adjustment was affected by fewer types of conflict than that of girls, suggesting that girls may be more responsive to family relationships generally, or more distressed by conflict between their parents.

There were also important differences in relationships between parental conflict and adjustment among children whose parents had settled the divorce by Time 2 in comparison with those whose parents had not. Children whose parents had settled the divorce showed almost no effects of either earlier or concurrent parental conflict at Time 2. In contrast, children whose parents had still not settled the divorce showed negative effects of earlier and concurrent violence or threats of violence.

Mothers' adjustment was somewhat related to parental conflict, particularly legal conflict involving motions regarding support and visitation. Mothers' adjustment was not, however, related to any indicators of aggressive conflict. Perhaps mothers who had experienced aggressive conflict blamed their husbands instead of internalizing, and they may have been relieved to escape this type of conflict. Divorce settlement acted as a buffer against the effects of parental conflict for mothers. Mothers whose divorces were still not settled at Time 2 were in worse shape if their divorces involved a large number of legal motions regarding children (i.e., if there were custody battles or disputes over support and visitation). Like their children, then, these mothers were affected by conflict related to their postseparation living arrangements, which were still in transition.

Perhaps reflecting male sex-role socialization that normalizes conflict, fathers' adjustment was unrelated to any type of parental conflict. We did find, though, that fathers whose divorces had been settled by Time 2 had fewer illnesses than those whose divorces had not.

Several characteristics of individual parents, families, and couples were associated with different levels and types of conflict. Spouse blaming, and high power motivation combined with low responsibility, were personality factors associated with higher levels of conflict. In addition, the gendered structure of the household—that is, the relative economic status of husbands and wives—in the period preceding the separation affected parental conflict. Couples in which the husband's job status was higher than that of the wife had lower levels of conflict than couples who had equal job status or in which the wife's job status was higher. Wives with greater earning power relative to that of their husbands have been found to be more likely to divorce than those with less earning power, as they are in a better position to support themselves and their families. In our sample, these mothers may have been more willing to engage in conflict than those with less earning power, who were more financially dependent on their spouses. Alternatively, the reversal of gender norms in their households may have provoked conflict.

Finally, couples who were able to cooperate in matters concerning the children, both before and after the separation, had lower levels of all types of conflict than those who were not. It is, of course, difficult to interpret the direction of causality in these relationships. Overall, we are struck by the importance of various kinds of conflict, particularly to children's adjustment, in the period following parental separation. The next chapter examines interaction patterns that maintain or restrain parental conflict in a small number of couples.

NOTES

1. Coding of conflict in the parental dyad was completed by coders who also coded conflict in other family dyads, without knowledge of the coding of other variables. Coding definitions and judgments were discussed until raters attained interrater reliability above .85; random spot checks of coding were performed to ensure that reliability was maintained at or above this level.

2. At Time 1, $r = .27$, and at Time 2, $r = .24$; $p < .01$ for both.

3. In order to determine whether couples who had settled their divorces by Time 2 had lower levels of conflict than those who had not, we assigned a code of 1 to couples whose divorces had not been settled and a code of 2 to those whose divorces had been settled by Time 2.

4. For legal motions related to children, $r = -.20, p < .05$.

5. $r = .39, p < .05$.

6. $r = -.20, p < .05$.

7. Regression analyses in Chapter 5 indicated that interpersonal conflict *was* related to mothers' adjustment at Time 2. This moderate effect emerged only in the regression analyses, in which four predictor and two control variables were also present. Thus, interpersonal conflict did have an effect on mothers' adjustment, but the effect was relatively small and only emerged when relationships with other variables were taken into account.

8. $r = -.55, p < .01$.

9. Spouse blame and self-blame were defined as the number of separate reasons for the divorce described by parents in the Time 1 interviews and attributed to the spouse and to the self, respectively.

10. TAT stories were scored for power motivation as described in Chapter 5 and for responsibility using the scoring system described by Winter and Barenbaum (1985) by coders achieving and maintaining a reliability of at least .85 with expert scoring. The responsibility scoring system includes imagery related to moral standards, obligations, concerns for others and for the consequences of actions, and self-judgment.

11. For verbal reasoning, $t = -2.00, p < .05$; for violence, $t = 4.02, p < .001$; for reports of husbands' violence, $t = 2.11, p < .05$; for Time 1 legal motions, $t = 2.13, p < .05$; for Time 1 interpersonal conflict, $t = 2.58, p < .05$.

12. $t = 2.49, p < .05$.

13. For comparison of verbal reasoning among fathers high in both power motivation and responsibility with other fathers, $t = -2.25, p < .05$. For correlation between responsibility and verbal reasoning among all fathers, $r = -.56, p < .05$.

14. Previous marriage was coded 1 if neither spouse had been married before, 2 if one or both had.

15. Correlations are with number of years of marriage before birth of first child.

16. Coparenting was coded 1 = poor, 2 = good. Our usual coding practices (2 years mixed together, coders "blind" to other data) were maintained; interrater reliability was maintained above .85.

17. Correlations are with mutual plans, coded 1 = no, 2 = yes.

CHAPTER 9

Patterns of Conflict and Parenting in Divorcing Couples

We have seen in several previous chapters that parental conflict has negative consequences, perhaps especially for children. Many parents in our study were aware of this; when asked at the end of the interview about advice they would give to other parents in the process of separation and divorce, most included warnings about not fighting in front of the children and about not dragging them into the conflict. Nevertheless, the stories and descriptions shared in the interviews demonstrated that the conflicts that motivate couples to divorce were not easily muted. We looked more closely at conflict within the parents' relationships by examining interviews with 22 couples in our sample. We used these data to try to identify the processes by which divorcing couples either maintained or contained their conflict; we also examined the implications of differences in this process for children's adjustment.

TWO PERSPECTIVES ON THE CONFLICT
IN PARENTS' RELATIONSHIPS

Because we wanted to understand something about the parental relationships, we focused only on the subsample of 44 men and women (22 couples) who were divorcing each other, and in which both partners participated both years. Although this is a small group, we wanted to get both points of view on

This chapter was drafted by Nia Lane Chester and Abigail J. Stewart.

the conflict, in the hope of obtaining a full and balanced portrait of couples' postseparation relationships and interactions.

We began by selecting two couples who described themselves as characterized by high levels of conflict. We compared these couples with two couples who were characterized by a relatively low level of conflict. Two of us[1] read Time 1 and Time 2 interview transcripts from these high- and low-conflict couples. As we read, we attempted to identify themes that captured differences between the pairs of couples and to go beyond either stylistic differences (e.g., dealing with disagreement by yelling rather than discussion) or merely demonstrating the different degrees of conflict in the couples (e.g., more "scenes" in the marriage histories of high-conflict couples). For purposes of consistency, we focused on specific sections of the interview, including reasons given for the separation; the nature of and satisfaction with current arrangements regarding custody, residency, and financial support; the nature of the couple's current relationship; ongoing areas of disagreement; and what things the parents perceived the child(ren) to be finding it hardest to adjust to. We also noted what the couple's children had to say about their parents' current relationship.

We then compared and discussed the themes; we agreed on a "consensus" set of six themes, described below. Each of us then separately applied these themes to a new set of pairs of high- and low-conflict couples. We discussed and compared our decisions, adjusted the themes a second time, and agreed upon a final scoring system. We then independently coded the interview transcripts from the rest of the couples with the final version of the coding system.[2]

DIMENSIONS OF CONFLICT

Six themes or dimensions captured differences between the "extreme" groups (i.e., the particularly high- and particularly low-conflict groups). These themes fell into two general categories: those involving the capacity for distancing or perspective taking, and those involving the ability to separate the parenting relationship from the marital relationship. With regard to the capacity for perspective taking, or distancing, couples differed in the following four ways:

Discrepancy in Accounts

The partners in high-conflict couples were more likely than those in low-conflict couples to give accounts and explanations of the divorce that were very different from each other. Their accounts differed not only in emphasis, but in content. For example, in one high-conflict couple, the ex-husband described long-running fights over the way his ex-wife had handled their money, saying that she had emptied out their bank account so many times before the separation that he'd taken her checkbooks away. His ex-wife, on the other hand, said that they had never fought over money. Discrepancy was particularly common in cases where violence was involved because the people alleged to be violent rarely mentioned their violent behavior in their accounts. One woman described terrible scenes in which she was beaten by her husband in front of the children and several occasions when the police were called; her ex-husband never mentioned any instance of violence.

Blame

Members of high-conflict couples tended to blame each other for the problems that led to the separation and divorce. Low-conflict couples expressed little blame of each other, instead using terms of mutual responsibility ("We just grew apart," "We just lost the ability to be happy with each other").

Empathy

The low-conflict couples seemed aware of each other's feelings and expressed some understanding and sympathy for the situations of the other. In contrast, the individuals in the high-conflict couples maintained a hostile stance toward each other, seemingly unable to see the ex-spouse in any context other than his/her role in the divorce. For example, one man, when asked about the reason for the divorce, stated, "She's a selfish bitch. She's breathing. That's the reason." This extremely hostile posture is reminiscent of a study by Johnston et al. (1989), in which clinicians describe how highly conflicted couples continue to engage in "negative ideation," casting their "ex" in stereotypically negative terms as a defensive way of "explaining" the divorce.

Avoidance of Conflict

In contrast to high-conflict couples, individuals in low-conflict couples described conscious efforts to minimize conflict by avoiding inflammatory topics or situations. This is not to suggest that they did not have strong disagreements with their exspouses. However, they were less concerned about making the other person change or admit blame. One woman in a high-conflict couple commented, for example:

"I'm not careful any more with my wording. I really don't care. If I end up arguing with him, I end up arguing with him. I will tell him exactly what I think and not let him intimidate me. Last night he said something about 'if the kids lived with him,' and I just said, 'Over my dead body.' I'm not letting him get to me."

This attitude contrasts with that of a man from one of the low-conflict couples. After describing a fight that involved his ex-wife's anger at hearing he had paid more attention to his girlfriend than to his kids on a weekend at the beach, the husband was asked by the interviewer how he had responded to his ex-wife's criticism. He replied, "I got defensive about it—we probably went around the loop for maybe 20 minutes or so—supposedly on that issue. We left it to be settled another time, and it has never come up since." His ex-wife commented about this same incident, "He assured me they [the children] had been well taken care of. What the truth of the matter is I don't think anyone really will ever know. Actually, I suppose it was probably somewhere in between perfect child care and the total 'lack of' story that I reacted to." This story reveals, in addition to conflict avoidance, how high- and low-conflict couples also differed from each other in their ability to separate their conflicted marital relationship from their relationship and functioning as co-parents.

The separation of parenting from the marital relationship was expressed in two more dimensions:

Coparenting Relationship

The low-conflict couples made a conscious effort to coparent, usually through frequent communication about the children. Decisions about the children were often made in collaboration with each other, although low-conflict parents were also likely to defer to the other parent's right to make decisions about the children when they were with that parent. "Whatever he does with them when they're with him is his business," one mother of a low-conflict couple commented, implying not only an acceptance of the father's right to parent, but also trust in his ability. Where there were disagreements, low-conflict couples were usually able to resolve them without resorting to personal attacks and with some understanding for the other's position. For example, when asked about parenting conflicts, the mother in the above-mentioned couple said:

"I sometimes think he should discipline them more. I've told him that. And he says he feels like the heavy. He has them such a short period of time he doesn't want to be jumping on them. I can understand that too.

But then when I get them I usually have some discipline problems be-cause they've been running amok. So we're working towards some mid-dle ground."

Parents in this group often were able to use common parenting "in-sights" as a way to be positive about each other. One woman described how her husband had been so critical of the children's eating habits that the din-ner table became a battleground and she began to eat in the kitchen. "But now that he has the kids," she said, "he's loosened up quite a bit and doesn't get so uptight about the unimportant things. He now sees that it's better not to serve the kids peas than to serve them and fight about their eating them."

In contrast, high-conflict couples were likely to be very negative about the other's parenting. All of the high-conflict couples in the "extreme" group identified at the beginning of the coding process were or had been involved in bitter custody or support disputes. In some cases there was evidence that con-cern about a particular parent's competence was legitimate, given past history of abuse and/or alcohol-related problems. Nevertheless, in only three couples did both parents seem intent on keeping every interaction hostile. As one boy in this latter group noted about his parents a year after the separation, "It seems like whenever they get a chance, one starts an argument, then the other keeps it going."

Creation of a New Relationship with Ex-Spouse

Low-conflict couples all articulated their awareness of the need to work out a relationship with each other that was different from their marital one, but that allowed them to continue to relate to each other as coparents. In some cases, the focus was on a new kind of connection: "We're not intimate friends," one father commented, "but we're more than just acquaintances." In other cases, the focus of this new relationship seemed to be on letting go of certain aspects of their old relationship. Commenting on the "narrowing" of their conversations, one man said:

"I certainly haven't asked for [my ex-wife] to be interested in how I'm doing, because I feel strongly that we can no longer worry about each other in *that* [his emphasis] way. We've got to be concerned about how we each together are going to meet our responsibilities to the children. We both feel that strongly. But we can no longer worry about how the other person is succeeding or not succeeding in life. Because each of us has to be independent of that concern because we are broken off in that respect."

In contrast to this effort to see each other in new ways, high-conflict couples seemed unable to see each other in any way other than as combatants.

CONFLICT MANAGEMENT TYPES

The focused comparisons used to develop these categories gave us some insight into some key differences between high- and low-conflict couples. After coding all of the couples in terms of the six dimensions, we were able to classify the 22 couples into three groups and explore patterns of relationship within these three groups in more detail. We were particularly interested in conflict management styles and the process by which some couples shift from a focus on disconnecting from each other as spouses, to the task of maintaining their connection as parents. We note that Ahrons (1995) studied a larger sample of men and women married to each other and made a similar effort to create a typology of conflict styles. Her sample was already divorced, included parents of minor children of every age, and was limited to couples in which the father was very involved in frequent visits with his children a year after the divorce. Moreover, her interviews covered somewhat different issues, she had no direct reports from children, and she did not apparently create the typology on the basis of systematic coding of themes. Despite these differences, the results of our two independent analyses are quite similar.

When we examined the pattern of couple scores (summarized in Table 9.1), it seemed to us that seven couples scored high on the conflictual end of the six dimensions. We thought of them as "battling," because most were openly hostile to each other.[3] Four couples scored on the other end of most of the dimensions; we thought of them as "allied," or at least as having achieved some kind of working truce.[4] The 11 couples in the middle were defined as "negotiating," although there was considerable variation in this middle group.[5] Some of them engaged in a good deal of blaming, but also showed some empathy for and willingness to work with each other around parenting. Others still seemed unwilling to cooperate with each other, but at least one parent was beginning to work on inhibiting the expression of conflict. A more detailed look at these groups illustrates these differences.

Battling Parents

Looking at the seven couples who represent the most extremely contentious group is helpful in understanding something about the way in which conflict is maintained, as well as the mechanisms by which its effects are passed on to

TABLE 9.1. Conflict Management Types

| Couple No. | Negative dynamics | | Positive dynamics | | | |
	Discrepancy	Blame	Avoid conflict	Empathy	New relationship	Coparenting effort
			Allied parents			
1			×	×	×	×
2			×	×	×	×
3			×	×	×	×
4			×	×	×	
			Negotiating parents			
5	×		×	×		
6		×		×		
7	×			×		
8		×	×		×	×
9	×	×				×
10	×	×	×			×
11	×	×	×			
12	×	×	×			
13	×	×	×			
14	×	×	×			
15	×	×	×			
			Battling parents			
16	×	×				
17	×	×				
18	×	×				
19	×	×				
20	×	×				
21	×	×				
22	×	×				

the children. These couples were not particularly similar to each other in terms of economic or educational backgrounds; they were, however, similar in the ways that they maintained negative interactions.

In many ways, these couples seemed still to be in the throes of what Bohannon (1970) called the "emotional divorce." Their feelings toward each other were characterized by intense anger; their interactions were tense, at best, and often quickly degenerated into heated arguments. There were few examples of interactions that were not divorce related. Ironically, the ex-spouses seemed intensely connected to each other in the passion of their negative feelings. In half of these couples, at least one of the partners mentioned "hating each other's guts." Many blamed the problems they were experiencing with their ex-spouses on their spouse's anger and hostility. "I can't get two words out without her starting in on me, bitching about this or that. I just hang up on her," said one man. His ex-wife observed in her interview that "he just gets angrier and angrier. He's impossible to deal with." Although at least one member of three couples assumed that their ex-spouse would like them to "drop dead," "get killed in an accident," or "disappear off the face of the earth," only one of the ex-spouses actually expressed this desire.

Given the difficulty with which these couples communicated with each other, it is not surprising that most were involved in legal actions beyond the initial divorce filing, but before the final divorce settlement (e.g., for temporary financial support, changes in temporary visitation schedules, and sometimes injunctions to keep one spouse away from the other, or the children). They tended to see the courts as a way to get for themselves what they believed they deserved, rather than as a way to mediate disputes. Yet they also frequently expressed bitterness about the legal process, the opposing lawyer, and their own treatment. "I wouldn't go across the street to save her lawyer from drowning," one man commented. Another observed bitterly, "If there was ever any hope that we could have come out of this thing having any respect or feeling for each other, the court system managed to destroy that very thoroughly."

Again not surprisingly, this group was the most likely to involve their children in their spousal struggles. Some did this directly, as in the case of a couple who split the custody of the children. Each believed the child living with the other parent was being turned against the noncustodial parent. Indeed, the relations between each child and the noncustodial parent were strained, as were the relations between the siblings themselves. The mother described a scene in which the father, against her wishes, went through the house taking things he wanted ("almost like a thief," one child commented).

Most of the other high-conflict couples also mentioned dramatic scenes that continued to take place in front of the children, or ways in which they made their negative feelings about the other parent known. One mother talked about how her continuing anger at her ex-husband made it hard to talk to her daughter, because she didn't know how to avoid saying "her father's a louse." She said she was careful not to criticize him in front of the girl, because "that kind of thing is so destructive." In the next few minutes, however, she described an argument she had with the girl's father about whether the 12-year-old should be allowed to be home alone after school: "I told him he should have showed a little interest before, and since when did he become the big expert. I said, 'When she's with me, it's none of your business.'" When asked if the girl was present during this argument, she said yes, but that she didn't think she was listening.

Some of the parents in this group more openly tried to engage the children as their allies in the "battle." One mother commented:

> "It upsets the boys when I've had an argument with him [her ex-husband], or I say, 'That son of a bitch, he ticks me off.' And [her son] will say, 'You shouldn't say that in front of us.' I'll say, 'You've got to know what he's really like. Believe me, you don't know the half of it.'"

In another case, the father rarely adhered to the visitation schedule, sometimes not seeing the children for a month at a time. The mother then planned a vacation with the children and wouldn't tell her ex-husband where they were going. He systematically took each child aside and tried to find out where the vacation was to be, with no success.

Most of the children of these warring families reflected their parents' conflicts. In all of the high-conflict families, at least one child was described as having difficulties with one parent or the other. Visitation was often problematic: In two families, one child refused to go; in two others, the children were described as "off the wall" and fighting among themselves upon their return; several parents described angry scenes that usually occurred at the point when children were being dropped off or picked up.

Children from three of the families were described as having had psychological difficulties before the separation (including "mild thought disorder," suicidal thoughts and gestures, and aggressive behavior), which had improved somewhat after the separation. In all seven families the children described themselves and/or their siblings as upset and angry. Most described their parents as "not getting along very well," or as getting along worse than they had before. Some weren't sure how they were getting along because "they never talk" (this latter comment was made by a child whose parents described themselves as not fighting in front of the children, but as having lots of arguments over the phone).

In general, then, the high-conflict couples were similar to each other, and different from the other groups, in the intensity of their negative feelings toward each other, their difficulty communicating with each other, their lack of cooperation as parents, and their inability to shield their children from parental conflicts in spite of their stated desire to do so. Four of the seven couples remained extremely hostile toward each other over the first year of separation and were involved in relatively constant contact, including unresolved legal disputes. The other couples were less "hot" after the first year and had relatively less contact. Usually one parent in these latter couples described the relationship as at least sometimes workable, possibly moving toward what one mother characterized as a "cautious truce."

Allied Parents

The four couples who were located at the other end of the spectrum on the six dimensions presented a strong contrast to the "battling" couples. The relationship between the separating spouses, for example, was generally not characterized by intense negative feelings and ranged from extremely positive to "business-like." One woman said that, although initially she "hated his guts," her husband had now turned into "the older brother that I never had." Apparently they were quite comfortable talking to each other about their respective romances, having lunch together at least once a week, and occasionally spending the night together. "It was never this good when we were married," the ex-husband commented.

Another allied couple described each other as good friends; the woman mentioned being happy that her ex-husband had become involved in a new relationship that seemed to be working. He indicated admiration for her recent educational attainment. They did not spend private time together, however, and were less emotionally involved than the previous couple. The third couple initially described themselves as very good friends. At the time of the first interview they were still working at the same company and had lunch together once a week. "It's really comfortable," the man commented, "but we both know it may change if one of us gets involved with someone." A year later, he described the relationship as somewhat strained: He was engaged, and his ex-wife was living with her lover. The fourth couple were the least close, describing their relationship as "meager" and "business-like" at the time of the initial data collection, and "better, but we'll never be friends" a year later.

In spite of the differences in the way they related to each other on a personal basis, each of these couples showed evidence of effective coparenting. Again, however, there were noticeable differences in the way they related to each other as parents, reflecting to some extent the style of their "ex-spousal" relationships. The first couple mentioned above described themselves as in perfect synchrony as parents, each praising the other's parenting abilities. Although the mother had custody of the children, they still did a variety of activities as a family and, according to her, hardly ever disagreed about the children. "We'll always be together as far as the kids are concerned," she commented, adding that the fact that they got along so well together made parenting the children much easier.

The other couples also interacted effectively as parents, but not with the same degree of agreement. "He's a marvelous, marvelous father," one of these other mothers commented. "I just wish he'd see the children a little more." Her comment is particularly interesting in that the father had custody of the children and lived in the preseparation family residence. She arrived every day as the father was going to work and stayed through dinner until he returned. Although this couple disagreed on some issues (as all parents do), in most cases they were able to arrive at some compromise.

Cooperative parenting did not always involve as much overlap and interaction as in the couple just described. A third couple from this group presented an interesting contrast, in that they didn't really parent together. Sharing legal custody, the mother had the children 3 days a week, and the father the rest of the time (including weekends). While they admitted to knowing (and caring) little about each other's personal lives, they said they were able to talk about the kids. For the most part, however, they parented very separately. "I don't worry about the kids with him most of the time," she said. "I wish I knew more about what he does with them, but however he takes care of them when he has them is his business. . . . He does his parenting and I do mine." This comment is actually similar to that made by one of the women in the battling group, except that in that case, she was acknowledging her own right to parent, not that of her ex-spouse. This allied couple offered few examples of any interaction with each other, although two instances were described, involving children's medical problems, where they clearly worked together, sharing their observations of symptoms and getting appropriate medical care. "I know she gives the children good quality care. She loves them and they love her," the father commented. At another point, however, he observed that he and his ex-wife were currently in a conflict over money and that "she won't talk to me about it, she has her lawyer do it." Yet he acknowledged, "In a way that's good, because we get into real bad arguments when we talk about money."

What distinguishes this allied group, then, is not one particularly harmonious parenting style. Some acted as a unit, others more independently (similar to the two relationship styles identified by Ahrons (1995) as "Perfect Pals" and "Cooperative Colleagues," both of which were also found to allow for functional parenting). What seems most important is that in each case the children clearly had the experience of having two parents. In addition, while the children undoubtedly experienced each parent differently, the legitimacy of the children's relationship with one was not challenged or sabotaged by the other. Where conflicts did occur, couples in this group tended to discuss the problem, or at least mention it, and try for some resolution. This resolution sometimes resulted in a behavioral accommodation by one or both parents (as in the case of one couple where she made an effort to oversee the children's dental hygiene more assiduously, at her husband's request). In other instances it resulted in a reduction of negative affect. In the latter case, the conflict was acknowledged, but let go once it got sufficiently aired, as in the example mentioned above where the issue had been whether the children had been well enough taken care of on the vacation in which the husband's girlfriend was included. Recall that in this instance, after "going around the loop about it," the argument was "left for another time," and never came up again.

What seems important, then, is not necessarily denying conflict and negative feelings, but perhaps not exacting a final "pound of flesh" either. It may be equally important that in conflicts in this group parents take a somewhat critical perspective on their own behavior. In the incident just mentioned, for example, the ex-husband admitted that he "got defensive" and the ex-wife ironically acknowledged that she had been advocating a level of probably unattainable "perfect child care."

The allied couples thus acknowledged their conflicts but were able to keep them from defining their relationship as ex-spouses or as parents. Indeed, too much closeness in a divorcing couple may be difficult to maintain and hard for children to understand. By the second interview, the couple who seemed so connected to each other had begun to draw apart. The father commented at this time that he was feeling the need to see his ex-wife less, to get on with the rest of his life. "We'll always be close," he said, "but she needs to understand that we'll never be as close as we were." When divorcing parents spend a lot of unconflicted time together, children may be confused about whether they're really getting divorced, thus delaying the adjustment process.

The handling of conflict among these allied couples may, of course, be a reflection of their marital or individual styles, and thus not easily learned by divorcing couples with a long history of more overt expressions of hostility in their marriages. However, there did seem to be an element that might be fairly readily learned by battling couples: conscious recognition of the need to develop a new kind of relationship, or at least a new way of relating to one another. The process of actually doing this involved willingness to communicate about parenting, respect for the other's right to parent, and avoidance of tactics that would directly or indirectly sabotage the other's relationship with the children. The development of a new relationship may also make it easier for parents to interact with each other comfortably, but not in a way that makes the children feel either that they are still angry or that they should still be married.

Most of the allied couples consciously articulated their efforts to find new labels for their relationship to each other. "We're the 'formerly married, forever connected through the children,'" commented one father. One couple was still struggling to define their new relationship. They gave numerous examples in their interviews of working together on problems having to do with the children, in ways that accommodated each other's needs (e.g., they talked once a week about the children; however, she called him at work because he said his girlfriend didn't like his ex-wife calling him at home). But they did not seem to be able to communicate effectively in front of the children. At the time of the second interview, the two children in this family disagreed about how their parents were getting along. The older thought they were getting along better and didn't fight as much. The younger said they weren't getting along and didn't like to speak to each other very much. Although this discrepancy may be partly due to different experiences of the children, it may also be that the parents were still ambivalent about their new relationship and thus communicated mixed messages in front of the children. Nevertheless, the variation in warmth among the other allied couples suggests that, while it may be possible for divorcing couples to remain friends with each other, even a "unique kind of friend," friendship isn't necessary for effective coparenting to occur.

Negotiating Parents

Half of the couples' relationships in our sample lay somewhere between the small "allied" group and the somewhat larger group of "battlers." In some ways this middle group of 11 couples is harder to summarize; nevertheless, the variations within it may reveal more than do the other groups about the process by which a divorcing couple can achieve spousal disengagement while at the same time salvaging their parenting relationship. This middle group may include more ordinary examples of parenting, even in nondivorcing couples. Not all married couples are as positive about each other as the "brother and sister" couple in the allied group, nor do all, possibly even most, parents believe that they are "always together where the children are concerned." So what are the ingredients that seem the most necessary for functional parenting in a situation where the parents are in conflict with each other?

Variations That Facilitate Parenting

Although not scoring on the "positive" end of all of the dimensions in our coding system, more than half (six) of the couples in the middle group gave evidence of providing adequate parenting, in spite of their lingering conflicts. As in the allied group, they varied in terms of the intensity and the direction of their feelings toward each other. Three couples seemed to be able to communicate with each other about parenting and to cooperate in decision making about the children, in spite of having little empathy, understanding, or caring about each other.

One of these couples expressed considerable hostility, anger, and distrust toward each other. She described their relationship as "very bad—a minus 50 on a 1 to 10 scale!" "I hate her," he said at the first interview. "We talk as little as possible." Neither entirely trusted the other's parenting skills (he felt he had done most of the child care during the marriage and was closer to the children; she felt he was too strict a disciplinarian). At the initial data collection they were in the middle of bitter custody litigation regarding the two children. They both exercised considerable restraint, however, in the expression of their concerns in front of the children. The boy had a close relationship with the father, and the mother said she did her best not to disrupt that and not to "pry" about the time spent with the father. She felt that her own relationship with the boy was good, although he was somewhat "standoffish" with her.

By the second interview, the custody of the boy had been awarded to the father. Both parents had sought counseling during this period. Although the mother was apprehensive about the custody arrangement, she accepted it, saying that she thought perhaps the boy would be happier with his father. Both the mother and the father agreed that their own relationship, while "guarded," had improved. What is striking about this couple is that, while there clearly remained underlying anger and hostility, they nevertheless were willing to communicate around parenting issues and to seek counseling about their differences in this area when their communication broke down. Although she was not entirely comfortable with the decision, the mother ultimately was willing to try a different custody arrangement with her ex-husband.

A different example of effort at coparenting in spite of lack of empathy for each other is provided by a family in which the father was relatively disengaged from the children at the time of the first interview. The mother felt that the divorce was mostly her ex-husband's fault, because of his drinking, explosive personality, and abusiveness (he stressed her religious views and personality differences). Nevertheless, she wished he would spend more time with the school-age daughter, whom he saw about once a month, according to the mother; according to the father, visitis were every other week. The mother also wished they could be more friendly with each other, because she'd feel better knowing he'd be available in a crisis.

At Time 2, this father was seeing his daughter more regularly (every other weekend and on several 2-week vacations) and was very positive about their relationship. He also mentioned that his relationship with his ex-wife was better than it had ever been, describing an incident in which they conferred about a problem the girl was having in school. The mother had argued that she should not be the one who always dealt with these problems and that he should talk to the teacher. He was at first uncomfortable with this idea, but eventually did talk to the teacher with, he felt, positive results. He felt more personally involved with his daughter's life, and the mother felt less burdened by taking on all parenting responsibilities.

It should be noted that the father had by this time joined Alcoholics Anonymous, was seeing a therapist, and had begun dating someone. The mother, on the other hand, was not sure about her future with the man she was seeing and was having more difficulties. However, she also felt that her relationship with her ex-husband was better, focused almost entirely on topics having to do with the child, with whom she agreed he had a "much improved" relationship. The child concurred, saying at the second interview, "We all get along good. They [her parents] don't yell at each other anymore." Interestingly, the older teenage child agreed about the improvement in the parents' relationship, but attributed it to the mother's new willingness since the separation to "stand up to" the father.

Although the mother in the above case saw herself as never having loved her ex-husband and described him in extremely negative terms, there was little overt hostility expressed on either part, and they clearly had improved in their ability to communicate about the focus child. In addition, real issues existed regarding the father's inappropriate behavior during the marriage, which he showed some willingness to address after the separation by entering therapy and joining Alcoholics Anonymous.

However, even ongoing negative feelings do not necessarily preclude effective parenting. For example, in another case where coparenting coexisted with negative affect, the father blamed his ex-wife and the women's movement for the dissolution of their marriage and had neither interest in nor sympathy for her efforts to develop a career. He described their relationship as "clerical" and as one in which communication was kept to a minimum. However, each parent was committed to the children's welfare: The woman noted that the man's girlfriend made life more "homey" for the kids; he was quite willing to increase his support payments in order to make it possible for the two children to attend a private school. Their ex-spousal relationship was business-like, not quite tense, and clearly based on their tacit assumption that each was willing and competent to make decisions in the best interests of the children.

These examples demonstrate that ex-spouses can function appropriately as parents even when they have little empathy or caring for each other. What seems important is the ability to contain their negative feelings within the arena of their ex-spousal relationship; this may be easier in situations where the blaming and discrepant accounts are focused on issues not having to do with the children.

Sometimes, understanding and acceptance of the other parent's limitations (whether real or assumed) can create an atmosphere that allows for effective parenting to take place, even though this may not entail any cooperative efforts between the parents. In two cases, one parent saw the other as having a major "problem." However, they did not let this perception negate the other's rights as a parent. For example, one couple was divorcing primarily because of the father's diagnosed mental illness and the mother's unwillingness to live with him any longer. Although not currently hospitalized, the father spent little time with his son and was not able to answer any of the interview questions about what his son was like. The mother, while showing some sympathy for her ex-husband's mental state, mostly expressed regret that he was incapable of being an effective parent. Nevertheless, she encouraged her son to visit the father regularly. The son was aware of his father's illness and seemed to accept the divorce and his father's inability to behave "like other fathers."

In another case, the parents were divorcing, by both of their accounts, because of the woman's relationship with someone else. The father had custody of the two children. Both parents had concerns about each other's parenting ability, however. For example, the father complained the mother was too lenient, and he worried that the children might be influenced by the "razzle-dazzle" of the mother's lover. At the same time, he expressed some sympathy for the mother's problems. The mother felt she had to correct for the father's somewhat oppressive lifestyle by being a little "frivolous" (by which she meant allowing the children more independence, taking them on outings, and allowing them more freedom in their choice of clothes and activities). She also expressed some sympathy for the father's loneliness and avoided criticizing him openly to her children. While this couple remained critical of each other's lifestyles and parenting and certainly did not parent together, they did not interfere in each other's lives. The children seemed clear about why their parents were divorcing and equally comfortable in both households. Here, then, as in the previous example, the presence of empathy, or at least acceptance, facilitated the parenting the children received, even if it did not involve parents conferring in a cooperative way.

Curbing Conflict in Hostile Relationships

What about the couples who remained hostile to each other, who felt no sympathy or allegiance to each other or to their connection as parents? Although like the battlers in most ways, the remaining five couples in the "negotiating" middle group were distinguished by at least one of the parent's efforts either to avoid situations likely to produce arguments or to inhibit consciously the expression of angry feelings. This was done with varying degrees of success, and it often occurred in families in which efforts were at the same time being made to enlist the children against one or the other parent. Nevertheless, the effort of even one parent to lessen the opportunity for the overt expression of conflict can be the beginning of a process that may lead to a more positive experience for the children.

Most of the examples in this group were of one parent trying to avoid conflicts with the other parent in order to minimize the effects on the children. For example, one mother, whose ex-husband refused to speak to her except through a third party and routinely criticized her in front of her son, said:

"I get very angry, but I hold my tongue. Because I know that if I say something to him, he'll know it aggravates me, so he'll do it all the more; so in order to save my son some grief, I just don't say anything."

This same mother said that she was careful not to confront her ex-husband with information she had learned from her son. On the other hand, she also felt that she needed to support her son, who, she said, hated being with his father. She described her son as having been "severely depressed" before the separation and as having improved "100%" now that the father was out of the house. She supported for the most part the highly structured visitation schedule established by legal agreement; when the father cancelled a visit, however, which happened fairly often, she refused to push the son to "make up" the time.

Another mother explained that things were better at the time of the second interview because she avoided settings where she and her ex-husband were likely to argue in front of the children. For example, when she knew he was coming to pick up the children, she waited outside with them, thus eliminating the fights that invariably seemed to occur inside the house.

A third example was provided by a mother whose relationship with her ex-husband was highly conflictual; during the first interview, she admitted to criticizing her husband openly in front of the children. During the second interview, she said:

"I used to outwardly act upset when he was late or would cancel out. . . . But I've learned not to open my mouth because it's something the kids have to deal with. . . . Instead of saying to them, 'Yeah, you're right, he's really a jerk, he was like that to me too,' I say, you know, 'I understand how you're feeling. You might try to tell your dad a little bit about how you feel.' So that's much more beneficial—so that he had to deal with their feelings. And they learn to talk to him instead of just complaining to me. He seems to listen to them more than he listens to me anyway."

It was striking that some parents felt that they had to strategize about how to present important issues without setting the other parent off. This was not always easy to do, however, particularly when a parent felt the safety of the child was at stake. For example, the mother in one of the more hostile but negotiating couples was angry about her ex-husband not providing their young son with appropriate safety equipment on his outings; she described at length her agonizing over how to present her concern to her husband in a way that would not start a fight, but would lead to his taking her request seriously. She eventually bought the boy safety equipment and markers to take with him to his father's house so he could decorate it as an "art project." She wasn't sure whether he actually ever used it, though.

The examples given above should be understood as occurring within a context that was not characterized by much cooperation among the parents. Most of the parents in the negotiating group were bitter about their ex-spouses and expressed this bitterness at least occasionally in front of the children. The efforts to inhibit expression of their negative feelings, however, were almost always described in the second interview, suggesting that, with time, some parents may begin to explore ways to defuse their hostilities. On the other hand, for some of these couples, as with the battlers, extremely negative interactions had been characteristic of their marriages and were likely to remain characteristic of their divorces. Nevertheless, the children of the negotiating couples were more likely than those of the battling couples to describe their parents' relationships as improved.

CONCLUSIONS

Data from our 22 couples suggest that the differences between divorcing couples who are battling and those who are allies are pervasive; it is easy to see how different their divorces must feel to their children. At the same time, the negotiating couples are striking in the range of relationships they are working out, different from both the battling and the allied couples. Despite the fact that our sample is small, it seems clear that many factors influence the kind of postseparation relationship couples can and do work out.

Although we feel confident that open war is not a constructive solution to continuing parental conflict, at the same time we hope to avoid idealizing any particular solution to the postseparation parental relationship. The individual temperaments and personal styles of the partners inevitably play a role in the kind of relationship that can be worked out; and some interaction patterns may be very difficult to change. In addition, the allied couples did not necessarily represent "ideal" dynamics. At least two of them may not have completed the work of altering their spousal relationships; their children may actually be confused by their relationship, and they may end up facing increased conflict as they eventually do separate. The couple in this group that was sharing custody managed their households quite easily; this might not be possible in families with more complicated household arrangements or more strained financial situations.

Nevertheless, one factor that clearly differentiated those couples who were stuck in their hostilities from those who seemed to be making some progress was the conscious willingness to try to manage the conflict, even if in only a small way. Even the most hostile of the negotiating couples described examples of actions they took to minimize the expression of their conflicts. The battling couples sometimes stated a commitment to inhibiting their hostile displays, but never gave examples of actually doing so.

A second important factor was the willingness to acknowledge the children's right to experience themselves as having two parents. This acknowledgment did not require warm relations between the parents themselves, but it did involve a willingness to support each other's status as a parent. Obviously this is a more difficult proposition in cases where there are legitimate concerns about the well-being of the child. Even in such cases, however, a parent can express concerns and seek limited contact with the parent in question in ways that avoid derogating that parent to the child.

Absence of conflict is thus probably less important than developing ways to manage the way it gets expressed. The couples who seemed the best at this were not necessarily less conflicted. They did seem less invested in their conflicts, however, and in some sense less interested in their ex-spouses, except as continuing partners, colleagues, or principals in a common parenting venture.

NOTES

1. Nia Lane Chester and Abigail J. Stewart.
2. Comparison of our results showed high agreement between our ratings; percent agreement = .90.
3. Ahrons (1995) labeled this group in her sample "Fiery Foes."
4. Ahrons (1995) defined a group that may have been like this as "Perfect Pals."
5. This group probably includes both Ahrons's (1995) "Angry Associates" and at least some of her "Cooperative Colleagues."

PART FOUR

PARENTAL DIVORCE AS A FAMILY TRANSFORMATION

In this final section, we consider the family as a whole. In Chapter 10, we assess the functioning of the family itself over time. We find that aspects of the custodial household are related to the mothers' adjustment in the early period, but much more strongly related to the children's well-being. We find, too, that aspects of the noncustodial household (like the children's relationship with their father) are important predictors of the children's adjustment. Most important, loyalty strains resulting from children being pulled betwen the custodial and noncustodial households are strongly related to children's adjustment at both times.

In addition to evidence that the family influences individuals' adjustment, we explore the relationships between custodial and noncustodial household functioning and the overall social integration of the family. We find that social integration is strongly related to the household's functioning, at least in the later period. This evidence suggests that by 18 months after the separation the new custodial household is functioning as a true "system" with new, loose connections with the noncustodial household.

In Chapter 11, we identify the key findings from our study and show how they are both consistent and inconsistent with folk wisdom about divorce. In this chapter we underline the value of viewing divorce as an event that affects a system of relationships rather than individuals.

CHAPTER 10

Families after Separation
CHANGING SYSTEMS

So far we have explored the experience of parental separation and divorce from the perspective of individual family members and of some of the dyads that make up families (mothers and children, and mothers and fathers). But we think of "families" as more than the sum of their individual members. In fact, families can be thought of as "systems," integrated units that link with other systems (schools, workplaces, neighborhoods, communities, etc.; see, e.g., Bateson, 1971; Bowen, 1978; Minuchin, 1974). When we think of families as systems, we notice that the whole system may be chaotic and disorganized, or rigid and routinized, even when we can't see any single individual in the system who either has those characteristics or imposes them on the family.

Family systems theory began with a model of families as having two married parents and children at home. Extrapolations to cover family structures that are different from that (childless households, gay and lesbian couple-headed households, single-parent households, etc.) are somewhat tricky (see Minuchin, Montalvo, Guerney, Rosman, & Schumer, 1967; Minuchin, Rosman, & Baker, 1978; Rice, 1994). Nevertheless, family systems theory is helpful in thinking about what may be going on in the course of parental separation and divorce because it makes clear that a unified system (which may have had serious flaws) involving two parents and children in one household is undergoing transformation into another kind of system, one involving two parents and children in two households, and, often, new adult figures related to the two parents, along with *their* children.

One question postseparation family members (like researchers) must come to terms with, then, is what *is* the postseparation "family"? Most often when there are minor children, a custodial household is created that includes

This chapter was drafted by Abigail J. Stewart.

a mother and all of the minor children. Sometimes this household also includes—constantly or occasionally—extended family members or a new partner for the mother. Is this custodial household, then, the "family"? A second,
noncustodial household is also created; in the dominant situation in our sample it always includes the father, sometimes includes extended family members
or a new partner, and intermittently includes the minor children of the marriage. Are these people part of the first family? Or an entirely different family?
In our view, the new, postseparation *family* includes two *households*. Ahrons
(1979, 1995; see also Ahrons & Wallisch, 1987) suggested the term "binuclear"
families to describe the phenomenon of families that have two "centers."

Interestingly, though, the nature of "binuclear" families is quite different
for different family members. In one-household families, all of the family
members can define their personal relationship to "the family" in the same
terms. In two-household families, different family members *must* define their
relationship to "the family" differently; it is, in fact, one of the central tasks of
separation and divorce for both parents and children not only to redefine, but
also to differentiate, their separate family situations. For the custodial mother, the family must now include only herself and her children (and maybe extended family or a new partner); though the noncustodial father may, in
some circumstances, remain a closely collaborating coparent and a resource
for her parenting, he is no longer part of *her* "family." At the same time, the
custodial mother must accept that the family for her children must include
both the custodial and the noncustodial household members. For the noncustodial father, there may be even greater confusion (and pain) in redefining

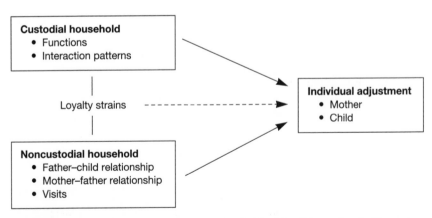

FIGURE 10.1. Family characteristics and individual family members' adjustment.
Note. Although fathers' adjustment may be a function of these same factors, the im-
portant predictors of adjustment for noncustodial parents deserve separate study.
Our sample of custodial father households was too small to permit parallel analyses.

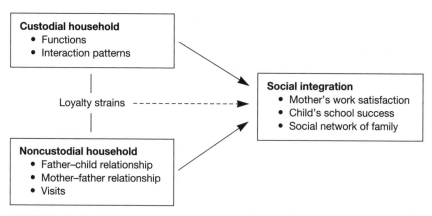

FIGURE 10.2. Family characteristics and the social integration of family members.

his household (if not his "family") as now including only himself on a daily basis, while his ex-wife and his children share a more populated daily household. Finally, children must accept the redefined family structure as including two households and find ways to negotiate being a child member of both.

In this chapter we will explore the postseparation family in two ways. First we will consider how various aspects of two-household families affect individual family members' adjustment. As we can see in Figure 10.1, features of both households—as well as the loyalty pressures between them—may affect children's and parents' adjustment, and they may have different effects early and late in the separating process. In the second part of the chapter, we will consider the custodial household as a family system that itself may or may not be well-integrated into the surrounding systems of work, school, and community. As we can see in Figure 10.2, in this part of the chapter we will examine the features of custodial and noncustodial households that support or weaken the *family's* overall adjustment in this sense. In this chapter, then, we will consider the postseparation family both as an environment with features that facilitate or block individuals' adjustment, and as a system with or without positive connections to wider social worlds.

FAMILIES AND INDIVIDUALS' ADJUSTMENT

All families, however they are defined, are expected to provide certain basic functions, or to meet certain basic needs, for family members (see, e.g., Lidz, 1968; Parsons & Bales, 1955; Pringle, 1974; Talbot, 1976). Postseparation two-household families must find ways to serve these functions for both parents and children. Because the custodial household is where the largest number of members of the preseparation family reside, where those persons spend the most time, and where child rearing is a daily feature of life, it carries a special burden after the separation.

It is this household that all family members (including the noncustodial parent, usually) expect should meet the daily needs of the children of the marriage. These daily needs have been articulated in a variety of different ways in the theoretical and empirical literature on families, but we selected six aspects that have been frequently suggested as critical for children's well-being in families: material resources, safety, regular routines, companionship, cohesion, and openness to feedback. These family features, because of their daily importance, will be explored in terms of the custodial households of the families we studied. In addition, several features of the noncustodial household will also be studied. We assume that adult family members also need to have most of these needs met in their families. Finally, consistent with the emphasis in family systems models of family functioning, we will examine the interaction patterns of pairs of family members, as well as the mother–father–child trio that now operates across two households.

What Makes a Family "Good" for Its Members?

It may seem intuitively obvious that it is "good" for a family to have certain features and not others. Most family theorists and researchers have, for example, assumed that it is "good" to have regular routines and clearly defined parent–child role boundaries (with parents the clear authority figures in the household). Sometimes single-parent families have been described as functioning "less well" than two-parent families on precisely these dimensions. We wondered, though, whether some family characteristics that work well in a two-parent family context might be less adaptive in single-parent households (see Rice, 1994, on this point).

For example, perhaps regular family routines provide a unifying counterstructure to a two-parent household otherwise organized around the work, school, and social schedules of two adults and some children. In contrast, perhaps single-parent households *need* to be less routinized if the single adult is to manage the different schedule constraints associated with her work and her children's school and social lives. Similarly, it may be reasonable in two-parent families to draw a boundary between adult authorities (who are united by that authority, among other things) and children. In single-parent households, though, such a sharp demarcation might encourage children to take an oppositional stance toward the now solo adult. Instead, a more egalitarian decision-making structure may both keep the peace and provide the isolated adult with feedback, assistance, and alliance. In short, although some features of families seemed likely to matter in the same way in two-parent and one-parent households (e.g., material resources, safety), we thought it was likely that some factors that are thought to be beneficial in two-parent households might *not* be beneficial in one-parent ones.

Our focus in this chapter is on the most frequent family configuration in our sample: one household includes the mother and minor children of the marriage; the other includes the father and sometimes others, with visits from the minor children of the marriage. Because our sample of custodial father families was so small, we could not include them in this analysis of differences among custodial households. Our analyses depend on indicators of household characteristics that are created by aggregating or summing the judgments of several different household members. We will use these summed judgments to assess which overall family characteristics (whether reported that way by the individual or not) are important for some or all family members' well-being.

FUNCTIONS OF CHILD-REARING HOUSEHOLDS

Features of the child-rearing households were generally coded from various family members' interviews (Table 10.1 lists the six functions of the custodial household that were coded). In many cases, no standardized measures of these constructs exist. Although observation of families might yield a different sense of how the household functions, we hoped that detailed interview accounts, obtained from several different family members, would provide us with a good sense of the "inside" of the family, at least as family members understand it. Extensive quotations support the conclusion that indeed the interviews did accurately reflect family member's experience.[1]

Material Resources

All families are expected to meet the material needs of family members. The postseparation custodial household may have much less access to economic

TABLE 10.1. Characteristics of the Custodial Household

Functions	Interaction patterns
Material resources	Close versus distant
Safety	Degree of open conflict
Regular routines	Role boundary flexibility
Companionship	
Cohesion	
Openness to feedback	

resources than the preseparation family did, partly because it no longer includes the family member likely to have the greatest earning power. Although the fact of fewer resources in postseparation mother-custody households has been well-documented (see, e.g., Kurz, 1995), the implications of the reduction of resources for children's psychological well-being, or their mothers', is much less well understood. In the course of their interviews, custodial mothers were asked to describe their financial arrangements, and overall financial situation. Three variables were coded from answers to questions about the following: the earning capacity of the custodial parent[2]; the financial contributions of the noncustodial parent to the custodial household[3]; and the financial difficulties reported by the custodial parent (including dependence on welfare, food stamps, or other such programs and reported problems obtaining basic necessities, such as food, housing, and transportation).[4] These three indicators were combined to create an index of material resources of the household.

Safety

Families are traditionally viewed as "safe havens," in which all members are (or should be) free from fear of physical or emotional harm. In families experiencing high levels of conflict (which postseparation families may be), it may be difficult to provide family members with a sense of safety and security. Family members tended to discuss the issue of safety only when it was *not* present; thus, feelings of vulnerability or insecurity were explicitly mentioned at various points in the interview, but perhaps particularly when we inquired into individuals' "worries."

For example, family members sometimes expressed anxiety about family members' mental or physical health ("I worry about my sister because she can't handle things," or "I worry about my dad, he's so depressed.") or potential injury (e.g., "I worry about my brother because he's little and if there's a fire he won't know what to do."). Other times they expressed concerns about not having basic needs met ("What's worse is there's no ... heat and it's cold."), or about being hurt by another person's violence ("I got scared when my dad started yelling. He might hurt us."), or about another person's intense affect ("I get scared because my mom's always crying."). Sometimes family members just express vague, unexplained anxieties ("I worry about my mother never coming home," or "I have scary nightmares," or "My mom's scared of my dad."). The point, from our perspective, was not whether these anxieties were reasonable or not (many of them were), but that all of these expressions of concern indicated that to some extent that individual experienced the family as a place of vulnerability rather than safety and security.

Coders for this variable read the entire interview transcript for an individual and recorded instances of expressed concerns about his/her own or others' physical or emotional safety (including worries about injury, death, and violence).[5]

Regular Routines

Families provide a structure for everyday life (meals, bedtimes, activities) that can offer a sense of stability to all members. The absence of a structure may leave family members feeling anxious and anomic, but this kind of structure can also be too rigid and may be experienced by family members as oppressive. In other research (see, e.g., Hetherington et al., 1982), single-parent families have been characterized as less highly structured and "regular" than two-parent families, perhaps because of the difficulty of one person imposing a structure on the whole family. It is not clear, though, whether these less highly structured households are experienced by family members as unpredictable and chaotic, or if they are simply less routinized, or have more complicated routines, than two-parent households.

One mother described her family's schedule after school:

"The first group [of kids] gets home from quarter to 3 and the younger group usually get home about quarter to 4. The nights that I'm working, I spend their time organizing who's going where, playing with what friend, what's going on for supper. Maybe taking someone to basketball.... The younger one's in Cub Scouts, so I do pickups and deliveries and things. The nights that I'm home, we usually have a big meal. I help my little one with his homework if he has it. I'm not there two nights during the week. So I communicate by phone, organize things, and I go off to work."

Although this kind of complex family life might sound chaotic to some, she concluded, "It's good. Life is active." When she was asked to describe how the dinner hour works, she said:

"There's two different kinds of dinner hours. There's the dinner hours I'm not there. That's usually set up by me and my older child, and that can be very flexible. That might be, as opposed to sitting at the table, eating in front of the television. That's loose and that's what I call 'garbage meal'—pizza.

The nights when I'm home we eat around 6, it's a big meal. After dinner hour also encompasses immediately after eating, an hour of drum lessons for my middle one, who sits in the middle of the living room, plays [his instrument] while we all try to do homework and drink tea and stuff. It's good; the kids are good.'

Although this might *sound* busy and noisy, after this period, it's "bath time and shower time, and then we start the bedtimes." As she put it:

"It's a very organized structure. There's sort of a chart on the wall and everybody kind of knows their role and everybody really pulls together. The four of us do, working and trying to be happy . . . they all know what time everybody's getting their showers, what time bedtime is, and if there's an exception we discuss it."

The regularity and predictability of both individuals' and families' routines was assessed, in terms of both weekday and weekend schedules. To try to capture not only the absolutely rigid routines, but also those that are organized in some more flexible way, we coded them as absolutely *consistent* if they were, but as *predictable* if events either occurred at exactly the same time every day, or in a highly predictable pattern—for example, at 4 P.M. on Tuesdays and Thursdays; other days at 3:30.

Children's interviews were coded for references to the predictability of their weekday routines in terms of after-school child care arrangements (where they went and who was there), degree of structure of after-school time (unstructured, some structure, complex structure), and regularity of bedtime (completely unscheduled, some leeway permitted, regular time enforced). Children's weekend regularity was assessed in terms of the degree of structure of weekend time (none, some, complex). Parents' interviews were coded for adults' own routines (regularity of time getting up, work schedule, and having "personal time" at some point in the day, as well as the degree of structure of weekend activity), children's routines (getting up, bedtimes, and home-from-school times, as well as the predictability of the child's method of getting home), and family routines (regularity of daily family dinner time and dinner preparation arrangements, as well as some weekly family activity—e.g., church, going to the movies, eating out, etc.).[6]

Companionship

Families are sources of companionship and provide protection from feelings of loneliness and isolation. The loss of one family member from the household may make it difficult for all family members to feel that this need is being met in the postseparation household. In addition, mothers may feel particularly bereft of adult companionship, even though prior to the separation the amount of companionship they were able to share with their ex-husbands may have been limited. The quality of the companionship experienced in each dyad in the household (parent–child and child–child) was coded, and then an overall household companionship score created by summing these scores. Companionship was rated in terms of the degree to which dyad members described themselves as spending time together sharing specific joint activities (talking, playing board games, going for walks, playing ping pong, etc.).[7] For example, one child depicted the companionship in his family in his description of his mother:

> "She likes to play with us and bring us to the beach and the movies when we're free sometimes. And she takes us fishing and out on boat trips with her friends every once in awhile."

His mother said:

> "I like the times when I can spend time with both my kids. I like times I can spend separately with each of them. . . . I really enjoy days like that, that we can just to go off, and we're close, and he doesn't feel inhibited by other people being around."

Cohesion

Families can provide family members with a sense of unity and community, partly because family members may feel that they share a point of view about the world. In the absence of a sense of cohesion, families may feel unorganized, and individuals may feel isolated. On the other hand, if demands for family cohesion are too great, family members may feel pressured into an unnatural conformity. In the postseparation situation, when family members may feel different degrees of loyalty to the noncustodial household, a strong sense of cohesion may be difficult to attain or unhealthy to require. Reiss (1981; see also Olson, Sprenkle, & Russell, 1979) has argued that one of the most important determinants of family cohesion is a shared perception of family events. In the case of divorcing families, shared understanding among family members of the reasons for parental separation may play a part in maintaining family cohesion—whether it's helpful or not—during a period of family change. Therefore we assessed family cohesion in terms of shared understanding both of the reasons for the divorce and of the judgment about who was to blame for it.[8] One family with a very cohesive view of the divorce agreed that the problems were related to the father's behavior. The mother said:

> "I think that what caused the separation was his usual going out and drinking with the guys in the afternoon and coming home for dinner late, and I just got fed up and said, 'Out.'"

Her 9-year-old child said his parents decided not to live together any more because "when my dad used to go out late and stuff, my mother got mad because he stayed out a long time." His older brother reported, "They couldn't get along and they always got in fights. My mother asked my father to move out, so he left." In families with low cohesion, children often either could not describe *any* reason for the separation or sometimes described very vague ones ("They didn't get along," or "They didn't love each other anymore.") that did not correspond well with the mother's account.

Openness to Feedback

Families are supposed to meet needs for emotional support of all family members; in order for that to happen, family members must feel able to make their needs clear and to define situations in which needs are not being met (see Olson et al., 1979). Thus, family members must feel free to describe unmet needs and to articulate how the family is not meeting them; these articulations normally come in the form of complaints or criticism.

The only available data for assessing this variable came from the children's interviews. Mothers rarely described instances of their own or children's efforts to offer critical feedback on the family, but children did describe such instances. For example, in one case a child described an occasion when he was unjustly accused by his mother of malingering. He said his mother "thought I wanted to miss school, so she sent me to school anyway. And I got sick." He let her know that this was not okay with him! In other cases, children complained about parents' unavailability to them because they worked too hard (custodial parents) or lived too far away (noncustodial parents). Finally, some children complained about parents not providing clear explanations for confusing situations, or not understanding and supporting them in difficult times.

Each child interview was reviewed in its entirety and each instance was recorded when children described an effort to offer a critical perspective on their family. We view these scores as measures of the child's sense that the family system is open to complaint and criticism—that is, feedback. We cannot know whether the system is actually responsive to the feedback, though it seems likely that children would stop expressing their unmet needs if their expressions were entirely futile. Aggregate scores[9] were created by summing the total number of instances recounted by each child reporter.

FAMILY INTERACTION PATTERNS:
THE CUSTODIAL HOUSEHOLD

Families with very different interaction patterns can serve the six functions just described. Whether a family is characterized by warm, close relationships or cooler, more distant ones, it can provide safety, material resources, companionship, and so on. However, family interaction patterns themselves—such as warmth and closeness—have also been identified as playing a role in individuals' well-being (see, e.g., Minuchin et al., 1978). Moreover, single-parent families have been described as having different, perhaps less desirable interaction patterns than two-parent families (e.g., more often having ambiguous "boundaries" between the parent and child roles or more ineffective parenting; see Hetherington et al., 1982; Hetherington, 1989). However, as we indicated earlier, some of these differences may arise from the different circumstances of one- and two-parent households; thus, ambiguous role boundaries could be problematic in the latter (in which the parental dyad is defined in contrast to the children), but not in the former (in which the single parent must make some alliances with his/her children). Table 10.1 lists the three kinds of interaction patterns we assessed in the custodial household.

As has been described in Chapters 5, 7, and 8 for particular dyads, we assessed every household dyad in terms of the *degree of open conflict* (low, medium, high) and the *degree of closeness* (vs. distance) in it (close, neutral, distant). In this chapter, overall household scores summed the ratings based on each reporter about each dyad in the household.[10] Finally, because of its importance in the literature both about single-parent households and about dysfunctional two-parent families, we assessed the *degree of flexibility in parent–child role boundaries* (see Minuchin, 1974, 1984; Minuchin et al., 1975). Interviews were coded for any mentions of occasions when relationships in the family did *not* reflect traditional, hierarchical boundaries between parents and children (e.g., with parents making rules and constructing routines and children following them). These included hierarchical, parental (rather than peer-like) relations among siblings (e.g., one child puts another to bed); parent–child role reversal (e.g., "My daughter gives me advice on what to wear on dates."); and peer-like relations between parents and children (e.g., "We're a team."). Although traditionally clear, firm boundaries between parent and child roles have been assumed to be desirable, it is less clear that this is so in single-parent households. In these households, peer-like alliances may be comforting to both parent and child, and some degree of parent-like caretaking activity by children may be comforting to parents and empowering to children.

RELATIONSHIPS AND INTERACTION PATTERNS: THE NONCUSTODIAL HOUSEHOLD

Our information about the noncustodial household mostly came from the children (who are certainly primary reporters); in a few cases (e.g., about the visitation schedule) we only had the reports of the custodial parents (who generally had a limited view of the noncustodial household, but had full information about visit scheduling). For that reason we could not assess the functioning of the noncustodial household on its own terms (e.g., the regularity of routines or safety). We could, though, assess the relations between the noncustodial and custodial household, both in practical terms (arrangements for visits) and in terms of the relationships among family members across households. Table 10.2 lists the aspects of these relations that we were able to assess.

Key indicators of the *relationship between the noncustodial household and the custodial household* included closeness and conflict in the mother–father dyad (as described by all custodial household members); closeness and conflict in the relationship between the father and the focus child of the study (as described by all custodial household members); and frequency, regularity, and stress of arranging visits between the noncustodial parent and the children (reported by the mother). The dyadic relationship variables involving the noncustodial parent were coded as described for custodial household relationships.

The presence of any loyalty strains (see Chapter 7) among the mother, the father, and the focus child was recorded. Such relationships have been identified as problematic for children in two-parent families; parental pres-

TABLE 10.2. Relations with the Noncustodial Household

Mother–father dyad	Father visitation
Closeness versus distance	Regularity of visits
Degree of conflict	Frequency of visits
	Stress of arranging visits
Father–child dyad	
	Mother–father–child triad
Closeness versus distance	
Degree of conflict	Loyalty strains

sure for loyalty in divorcing situations has been seen as analogous to the kinds of triadic pressures that arise within "intact" households (see Minuchin, 1974, 1975, 1984; Minuchin et al., 1978). Loyalty strains, or triadic relations, were considered to be present when children reported themselves or were seen by others as "caught" or torn between conflicting loyalty to their parents; or when they directly tried (or were seen as trying) to manipulate or play parents off against each other. Loyalty strains were also coded when they were more clearly parent initiated, as when parents made (or were perceived to be making) direct requests for loyalty or expressed distress over a child's "disloyalty."[11]

One mother described a situation in which her son needed new sneakers and asked his father for them. His father said, "Have your mother buy them," and his son replied (accurately) that "she doesn't have the money." The father then suggested to the boy that his ex-wife's boyfriend could buy them. This kind of interaction obviously places the child in an impossible position in the middle of the parents' conflict with each other.

We asked the children in the family our usual question: "Sometimes after a separation, kids feel kind of caught. Like, if they say one thing it makes their mom mad, and if they say another thing it makes their dad mad. Does that ever happen to you?" The younger child in the family described above said, "It always does. Like when my dad calls here, my dad always wants to talk to my mom, and they get in a fight. And I'm on my dad's side and my mom's yelling because we're disagreeing with her." This boy's older sibling responded to the same question this way:

> "Like something you're not supposed to tell? Yeah. My mother has another boyfriend that she's been seeing for awhile, but he went back [to another state], and my father didn't know about it. And we made a mistake, and we thought he knew about it, and we told him. . . . And then he told my mother, and my mother talked to us about it, and so now we don't tell anything to the other person that one doesn't want to. That's happened quite a bit."

Clearly loyalty conflicts were a prominent feature of this family's interactions in the postseparation period.

Finally, the *regularity and frequency of visits* between the noncustodial parent and his children were coded on the basis of mother reports. Although we had asked children about these same issues, we found that their reports were quite vague; they did not seem able reliably to report about either regularity or frequency, often indicating that they saw their fathers "pretty often" or "not too much" rather than being able to identify a pattern. Mother reports of the frequency of visits were coded into four categories: never or only once since the separation, less than twice/month, two or three times/month, at least once a week. The visits were also coded as occurring on a fairly regular schedule, or not. At Times 1 and 2, visits were quite frequent, in that about two-thirds of the pairs visited at least twice/month. Most (two-thirds) of the visits at Time 1 were on a "regular" schedule; however, at Time 2, most visits were not regular (about two-thirds).[12]

As was described in Chapter 3, mothers also reported on the degree to which either making the arrangements for visits, or the actual visits themselves, were stressful for them or the children (about one-quarter found them stressful at Time 1 and about one-third did at Time 2).

INTERRELATIONSHIPS AMONG HOUSEHOLD CHARACTERISTICS

The different aspects of family functioning that we coded might not really measure separate features of family life. One indication of that would be a high level of intercorrelation among the variables. The custodial household variables were actually not highly intercorrelated; moreover, the correlations were not the same across years. The variables assessing relations with the noncustodial household were also not highly intercorrelated except for visit frequency and regularity (as mentioned earlier), and visit frequency and father–child closeness.[13] Therefore, we are confident that the different family variables assessed independent aspects of the custodial and noncustodial households.

CHANGE DURING THE POSTSEPARATION PERIOD

It seems reasonable to expect that family functions in the custodial household, links between the two households, and interaction patterns in the custodial household and with the noncustodial parent would change a great deal in the postseparation period (between 6 months and 18 months after the physical separation). However, most of these variables were actually fairly stable over time. Even so, there could be stability of families' relative levels on these variables, and at the same time all of them could be changing in one direction or another (thus, loyalty strains could be decreasing overall, but the various families could retain their same relative position compared with each other).

However, matched *t*-tests assessing change over time indicated that all but one variable showed no consistent pattern of change over time. The only one that did show significant change was the regularity of father–child visits (which decreased significantly). This overall lack of change may suggest that, within about 6 months after the separation, fairly stable patterns of interaction and household organization had been established.

CUSTODIAL HOUSEHOLD CHARACTERISTICS
AND INDIVIDUALS' ADJUSTMENT

Early postseparation characteristics may provide (or fail to provide) an important facilitating environment for individuals' adjustment at the time. It would be reasonable to expect that all household members would be more comfortable—better adjusted—in households that are described by household members as safe. On the other hand, some of the measured household features (e.g., companionship) may or may not be important factors in individuals' immediate adjustment, because there may be other important sources of satisfaction of that need (e.g., friends).

Similarly, some features (e.g., material resources) may be a more important factor in the adjustment of adults than children, whereas others may matter more for children. Finally, whereas some factors may matter in the short term, others might only be important over the longer term.

Features of the Family and Household
Members' Adjustment

In the next sections of the chapter, the relationships between features of the family (involving the custodial and noncustodial households separately) and mothers' and children's adjustment will be presented. These relationships were assessed by multiple regression analyses, in which a group of family characteristics was treated as predictors, and their separate relationships with individual family members' adjustment was assessed, while at the same time controlling for the other family characteristics.[14] Thus we can judge, for each type of family member, within each time period and over time, which family features were most important.

In addition, as in previous chapters, we examined the effects of the family characteristics for various subgroups.[15] For example, we assessed whether families that are both conflictual and experienced as unsafe are more problematic than families that are only one or the other. For children, we also considered the effects of the various family features for children of different ages and genders.

Features of the Family and Mothers' Adjustment

Table 10.3 summarizes the pattern of significant relationships between family features and mothers' adjustment within and over time.[16] Within Time 1, there was a significant overall relationship between the set of custodial household characteristics and mothers' psychological adjustment; material resources, safety, and openness to feedback were the critical features. These

TABLE 10.3. Predicting Mothers' Psychological Adjustment from Family Variables

Family variables	Significant predictors		
	Within Time 1	Over time	Within Time 2
Custodial household variables			
Cohesion		−	
Companionship			
Openness to feedback	+		
Material resources	+		
Regular routines			
Safety concerns	−		
Dyadic closeness			
Dyadic conflict			
Role flexibility		+	
Noncustodial household variables			
Father–child closeness			
Father–child conflict			
Mother–father closeness	+		
Mother–father conflict			
Ease of arranging visits			
Frequency of visits			
Regularity of visits			
Loyalty strains			

Note. + indicates a significant positive relationship; − indicates a significant negative relationship. Relationships depicted in this table are presented in detail in Appendix Tables 10.1 and 10.2

findings echo those reported in Chapter 5 suggesting that in the early period the mothers were especially preoccupied with the most basic functions of the new household—in this case, providing adequate material resources and safety. Nevertheless, it should be noted that interpretation of relationships within time is always tricky, because the causal direction might run either way (or both ways). Mothers who are better adjusted may be the heads of households that are experienced as safe, materially secure, and open to criticism. Alternatively, households that are experienced as safe, materially secure, and open may facilitate mothers' psychological well-being (either because their own needs are being met or because their children's needs are). Obviously, causal relationships could truly run in both directions.

Different Time 1 household features predicted mothers' adjustment over time: lower levels of early family cohesion and higher levels of role boundary flexibility were associated with Time 2 well-being. Especially in combination, these two characteristics seem to assess the degree to which the family atmosphere is relatively free and unconstraining.

When family cohesion was high, in our study, family members shared a view of the reasons for the parental divorce and blame attribution. This kind of shared view may be fairly inappropriate, or even oppressive, in a household composed not only of people at different developmental stages, but with different continuing relations with the noncustodial parent. For mothers and children to share the same view of the divorce, that view must be fairly simple and unsophisticated. This may happen when the reason for the divorce is in fact simple and evident—for example, when alcohol or violence is involved. Alternatively, it might reflect a mother's early postseparation need to press her children to share her view of the divorce and her ex-husband. Over time, in any case, collective adoption of this kind of simple (probably negative) view might well exacerbate tensions, leading to difficulties in working out comfortable visitation arrangements with the noncustodial parent.

It is interesting that just as a cohesive family view was not helpful to mothers' well-being, maintenance of rigid parent–child boundaries within the household also was not. Especially in the early postseparation period, insistence on rigid parent–child roles may preclude creative solutions to household logistical problems (Minuchin, 1984, makes a similar point). It seems clear that for mothers the important issue in the early period was the family's ability to meet basic needs, while over time freedom from a constraining family ideology (about roles or about the story of the divorce) may have permitted more open-ended problem solving.

At Time 2, characteristics of the later postseparation custodial household were unrelated to mothers' adjustment, suggesting that for mothers the importance of these characteristics was confined to the early postseparation period. However, it should be noted that concerns about safety in both the early and the later period affected the impact on Time 2 adjustment of both early family cohesion and later family openness. Thus, if there were many safety worries in the early period, early family cohesion was particularly strongly related to poor later maternal adjustment. This suggests that cohesion that *was* tied to negative family circumstances (producing safety worries) was indeed problematic. Additionally, in families with many safety worries at Time 2, openness to feedback was related to poorer mother adjustment. Thus, in families that felt unsafe, mothers' adjustment was worse if they could not distance themselves from children's critical feedback or different view of the divorce.

Finally, companionship, regularity of routines, dyadic closeness, and dyadic conflict were unrelated to mothers' psychological adjustment at both times. One possible explanation for this may be that these features of the custodial household actually were also features of the preseparation household. They may, then, have been experienced as "constants" and as irrelevant to mothers' adjustment. Alternatively (or in addition), perhaps these characteristics of the postseparation household are more in the control of the custodial parent and therefore do not affect her adjustment one way or the other.

In the bottom half of Table 10.3, features of the noncustodial household are listed. Because the mothers in these families had the most tenuous relationship with the noncustodial households, we expected few, if any, relationships between her well-being and family functions and interaction patterns in that household. Indded, as only one relationship emerged within or over time, it probably should not be interpreted.

Despite the lack of direct effects of noncustodial household characteristics on mothers' adjustment, the degree of conflict between mothers and fathers affected the relationship between these characteristics and mothers' adjustment. Thus, the joint presence of low mother–father conflict and high father–child closeness (as opposed to any other combination of these variables) was related to good adjustment for mothers over time. At the same time, when mother–father conflict was high, closeness in the father–child relationship was related to poor adjustment in mothers. These results illustrate well how one dyadic relationship can influence family members outside that dyad. Similarly, in the later period, fathers' visit regularity was associated with good mother adjustment, *if* the mother–father dyad was low in conflict. If the mother–father dyad was highly conflictual, on the other hand, visit regularity was associated with poor mother adjustment. Overall, then, conflict in the mother–father dyad, like other features of the noncustodial household, was not related to mothers' adjustment directly, but it did affect the impact of other features of postseparation family life.

Features of the Family and Children's Adjustment

Tables 10.4 and 10.5 summarize the relationships between family characteristics and children's self-reported and mother-reported adjustment within and over time.[17] Analyses of the impact of family variables on children's adjustment paralleled those for mothers, except that we also controlled for age and gender. (The direct effects of age and gender on adjustment were already discussed in Chapter 6.) Taken together, the set of custodial household features was most strongly related to mother reports of behavior problems, but there were also some relationships to children's self-reports of adjustment and mothers' reports of children's illness. Specifically, family cohesion and dyadic distance (vs. closeness) were associated with poorer adjustment according to children's self-report. Dyadic distance in the early period also tended to be related to poorer child adjustment in the later period. Not surprisingly, then,

TABLE 10.4. Predicting Children's Self-Reported Adjustment from Family Variables

Family variables	Significant predictors		
	Within Time 1	Over time	Within Time 2
Custodial household variables			
Cohesion	–		
Companionship			(+)
Openness to feedback			
Material resources			
Regular routines			
Safety concerns			
Dyadic closeness	+	(+)	
Dyadic conflict			
Role flexibility			
Noncustodial household variables			
Father–child closeness			
Father–child conflict			
Mother–father closeness			
Mother–father conflict			
Ease of arranging visits			
Frequency of visits			
Regularity of visits			
Loyalty strains	–		–

Note. + and – signs as in Table 10.3. (+) indicates a trend ($p < .10$) for a positive relationship; (–) indicates a trend ($p < .10$) for a negative relationship. Relationships depicted in this table are presented in detail in Appendix Tables 10.3a, 3b, 4a, 4b, and 4c.

close dyads in the custodial household supported children's self-reported adjustment, though a shared view of the divorce did not.

Few material resources, lack of safety, and household conflict were all associated with children's poorer adjustment according to mothers' reports (particularly of behavior problems). For children, though not for mothers, the effects of fewer material resources and a lack of safety persisted over time. The fact that lack of material resources and lack of safety also related to mother's own poorer adjustment in the early period may have amplified the impact of these variables, which do seem to index the postseparation family's ability to meet very basic needs.

Finally, conflict and regularity interacted with each other in the later period. Households characterized by high conflict and high regularity had children with higher self-reported adjustment and lower mother-reported illness than other households. Adjustment was also high (and illness low) in house-

TABLE 10.5. Predicting Children's Mother-Reported Adjustment from Family Variables

Family variables	Illness			Behavior problems		
	T1	OT	T2	T1	OT	T2
Custodial household variables						
Cohesion						
Companionship						
Openness to feedback						
Material resources				−	−	
Regular routines						
Safety concerns				+	+	
Dyadic closeness						
Dyadic conflict	(+)			+		
Role flexibility						
Noncustodial household variables						
Father–child closeness	−		(−)			
Father–child conflict		(+)				
Mother–father closeness						
Mother–father conflict	+					
Ease of arranging visits						
Frequency of visits						
Regularity of visits						
Loyalty strains				+	+	+

Note. +, −, (+), and (−) signs as in Tables 10.3 and 10.4. T1 indicates relationships within Time 1; OT indicates relationships over time; T2 indicates relationships within Time 2. Relationships depicted in this table are presented in detail in Appendix Tables 10.3a, 3b, 4a, 4b, and 4c.

holds in which both conflict and regularity were low. These results suggest that regular routines may serve a helpful organizing function in a household that is tense, but may feel oppressive in a household that is not.

Overall, many of the same features of the custodial household affected mothers and children. In particular, lack of material resources and of safety was problematic for both, while freedom from a shared view of the divorce was helpful. However, as we expected, but in contrast with findings for the mothers, noncustodial household characteristics had many direct and moderated relationships with children's adjustment in both the early and the later period.[18]

Perhaps the most striking finding is that loyalty strains were associated with poorer child adjustment, according to mother and child reports within and over time. In addition, lack of father–child closeness was associated with mothers' reports of children's illness at both times. However, frequency, and regularity of visits, and stressfulness of visit arrangements only showed complex relationships, depending on children's age and sex.[19] Boys and younger children were better adjusted when visits were more frequent, more regular, and described as less stressful to arrange. Surprisingly, girls and older children were better adjusted when visits were less frequent, less regular, and more stressful to arrange. This pattern of results may suggest that children with relatively stronger or more unambivalent needs for approval from their fathers (boys and younger children) benefited from more contact with them. In contrast, children who were more prepared to be independent, or who were more likely to feel divided loyalty (older children, and girls—who may be more identified with their mothers) did not.

Father–child conflict also had complex relationships with adjustment, depending on age and sex, especially in the later period. Boys in conflictual dyadic relations with their fathers showed poorer adjustment over time, while for girls it was being in low-conflict dyadic relations with their fathers that was related to poor adjustment over time. At both times, older children in nonconflictual dyadic relations with their fathers, while younger children in conflictual relations with their fathers, showed poorer mother-reported adjustment. This pattern, much like the pattern for visitation, suggests that boys and younger children responded negatively to high conflict with their fathers, whereas girls and older children actually responded negatively to low conflict. It may be that the conflict is actually qualitatively different for these different groups, or it may be interpreted differently by boys and younger children than by girls and older children. Establishing and maintaining a relationship with the father without having the mother present may feel very different to these different groups of children. Boys and young children may be particularly sensitive to the risk of rejection associated with conflict with their noncustodial fathers. Girls and older children may feel more comfortable with some distance in their relationships with their noncustodial fathers; for them, conflict may signal both connection and distance in a way that is tolerable.

Some features of the relationship between the noncustodial parent and the custodial household were generally important for most children. Thus, loyalty strains were problematic across the board, as was a lack of father–child closeness. However, the impact of other variables—particularly aspects of visitation and father–child conflict—depended crucially on age and gender.

What Did Matter for Individual Family Members?

We have seen, in this first part of the chapter, that mothers' adjustment depended most strongly on features of the custodial household at Time 1. During this early period, mothers' adjustment was facilitated by a certain degree of flexibility and openness, as well as by having basic material and safety needs met. Relations with the noncustodial household did not have much effect on her well-being, unless the mother–father dyad was conflictual. In that case, aspects of the father–child dyad and of the father's visit schedule were associated with her adjustment. By Time 2, even the characteristics of the custodial household had little impact on her well-being.

For children, the relationships were stronger, underscoring children's greater dependence on their households in getting their needs met. The most consistently problematic interaction pattern was loyalty strains between the custodial mother, noncustodial father, and the child. According to children's self-reports of their adjustment, and their mothers' reports of their behavior and illness, loyalty strains produced difficulty for children throughout this postseparation period.

Close dyadic relationships and conflict in relationships were also important predictors of children's adjustment at both times. However, conflict and closeness in the relationship with the father had different effects for children of different ages and sexes. Boys and young children were negatively affected by conflict, whereas girls and older children seemed to find such conflict helpful.

Finally, children's adjustment was particularly negatively affected by problems with basic needs in the postseparation household at Time 2. Perhaps children are sufficiently reassured by relational closeness in the early period that they can tolerate disruptions of these needs, but a year later difficulties around safety and material resources do jeopardize their adjustment. These findings suggest that social support for households headed by single parents—support that permits them to meet safety and material needs—may play a critical role both in mothers' early ability to adapt to their new family situation and in children's later adjustment.

THE FAMILY IN A WIDER WORLD

As was mentioned at the beginning of this chapter, postseparation custodial households can be characterized not only in terms of individual family members' adjustment, but also as having varying degrees of family-level "adjustment." Thus, family members may be viewed as more or less well-connected with people outside the household in a network of relationships, and as "successful" in the school (for children) and work (for adults) spheres. To create a measure of this kind of family adjustment, or *social integration*, we summed each *child's school performance* (as self-assessed[20] and as assessed by the mother[21]), the mother's self-rated degree of *satisfaction with her work life* (including being a homemaker), and each family member's degree of *integration in a social network* outside the custodial and non-custodial households.[22]

We expected that the overall social integration of the custodial household would be facilitated by some internal household functions and interaction patterns, and that relationships might be different for subgroups of families (high–low conflict, high–low cohesion, etc.). Table 10.6 summarizes the relationships we found.[23]

Although there were several trends, there were no significant relationships between early household characteristics and *early* family integration, though the relationships between these characteristics and both mothers' and children's individual adjustment in this period were substantial. The relationships with family social integration were somewhat stronger over time: dyadic closeness and low dyadic conflict (along with a nonsignificant trend for high cohesion) facilitated later family social adjustment. It is striking, though, that there were very strong relationships in the later period between family social integration and custodial household characteristics (in contrast with individual family members' adjustment, which was *not* strongly affected by custodial household characteristics at Time 2). Companionship, safety, openness to feedback, and (to a lesser degree) closeness were *all* associated with better family social adjustment at Time 2. In addition, conflict and lack of material resources moderated the relationships of a number of variables (including regularity of routines) and family social adjustment. Companionship and openness were especially beneficial in low-conflict families, while regularity of routines was most helpful in high-conflict families.

Some other features of the family were particularly problematic in combination; thus, the combination of conflict and worries about safety was relat-

TABLE 10.6. Predicting Family Social Integration from Custodial Household Variables

	Significant predictors		
Family variables	Within Time 1	Over time	Within Time 2
Cohesion	(−)	(+)	
Companionship			+
Openness to feedback	(−)		+
Material resources	(−)		
Regular routines			
Safety concerns			−
Dyadic closeness	(+)	+	(+)
Dyadic conflict		−	
Role flexibility			

Note. +, −, (+), and (−) signs as in Tables 10.3 and 10.4. Relationships depicted in this table are presented in detail in Appendix Table 10.5.

ed to particularly poor family social integration. Similarly, lack of material resources coupled with safety concerns in the later period was associated with lower integration than poverty alone. In contrast, although at both times household conflict and lack of material resources alone were both risk factors, it was not worse to have both. Finally, in the later period, family social integration was higher in households with more resources that had flexible role boundaries, and was lower in families with more resources that had rigid role boundaries. Families with more resources and rigid internal role boundaries apparently also maintained a firm boundary between themselves and other social systems, while similarly prosperous families with more flexible internal boundaries had more permeable boundaries with other social systems. It seems likely that families with rigid boundaries were using resources to maintain their self-sufficiency, while those with flexible boundaries were using them to link with the wider world. In poorer families, internal role boundary flexibility was simply less relevant to family social integration, probably because resources were necessarily directed toward more basic needs.

Interestingly, there were virtually no relationships between noncustodial household characteristics and custodial household social adjustment at either time (in contrast to the findings for children's individual adjustment). The single exception was that in the early period, less closeness in the parental dyad was related to better family adjustment; it was, though, also related to poorer maternal adjustment.

What Mattered for the Family's Social Integration?

There were few relationships between family social integration and either custodial or noncustodial household characteristics in the early period. There were, however, very strong relationships between custodial household features and social integration in the later period, suggesting that the household was operating as a tighter "system" at Time 2. All of the household characteristics except cohesion had strong effects, though conflict and material resources had only moderating (not direct) effects. The noncustodial household features did not seem to be relevant to the social integration of the custodial household (despite their strong relevance to children's psychological adjustment).

Each of the features of family life that we examined played some role in the adjustment of individual family members or the household unit. All of them, then, are important. But if we take a family systems perspective seriously, we needn't worry about how members of families with divorcing parents could attend to them all. Fortunately, in a system, attention to one factor (e.g., increasing material resources or dyadic closeness) will inevitably have implications for others.

CONCLUSIONS

Across the many different findings about the relationships between family characteristics and children's, mothers', and households' adjustments, what patterns emerge? We can consider this question both in terms of the consistencies that emerge across the different kinds of adjustment (mothers', children's, families'), as well as the specific predictors of each separate kind of adjustment.

Across the different kinds of adjustment, we have found material resources, a sense of safety, and dyadic closeness (both in the custodial household and with the noncustodial parent) to be factors that facilitate adjustment in the earliest period after separation. These factors involve the meeting of very basic human needs; it seems clear that a family environment that is meeting those needs is important to both mothers and children.

Characteristics of the early postseparation household that seem to have enduring consequences over the next year for mothers and children are different. For children, safety and security continue to be crucial; for mothers, flexibility becomes important over time, perhaps because of its value in their problem solving as single parents.

Finally, in the later period, the most important family features are the combination of conflict and regular routines. When household conflict is low, regular routines interfere with adjustment. However, when household conflict is high, regular routines support adjustment, perhaps because they help contain the conflict. At the same time, when conflict between the custodial and noncustodial parents is high, regularity in father–child visitation is problematic, perhaps because, in this instance, increased regularity provides regular opportunities for conflict, rather than containing it. This pattern of findings suggests, contrary to a great deal of advice they are likely to encounter, that single parents should not always strive to achieve a highly routinized household.

If we search for the family characteristics that matter for mothers' adjustment in ways that are *different* from the pattern for children, we find that for mothers role boundary flexibility is a more important factor in adjustment, as is the interaction of interparental conflict and father–child closeness. For mothers in conflict with their ex-husbands, closeness in the father–child dyad is difficult to accept; for mothers not in conflict with their ex-husbands, closeness in the father–child dyad facilitates adjustment.

The most striking factor predicting children's poorer adjustment (but not their mothers'), is loyalty strains; it was important early, over time, and later. There can be little doubt that this interaction pattern is detrimental to the adjustment of children after parental separation. In addition, both interparent conflict and household conflict were more important negative predictors of children's adjustment than of their mothers' or their families'. The significance of these factors is underlined by the fact that they predicted children's adjustment, regardless of age and gender. This is notable as age and gender were important moderators of the impact of several variables involving the linkage of the two households.

Some factors that were helpful to boys and younger children (notably regular, frequent, and stress-free visits with their fathers) were actually detrimental to the adjustment of girls and older children. Given the fact that all of the families we studied in this chapter had the same gender structure (female-headed custodial households, male-headed noncustodial households), it is difficult to know how the gendered family system may have influenced these findings. Only research on families with father-custody and noncustodial mother households could demonstrate whether boys would then feel more loyalty strain and girls would benefit from more frequent, regular visits with their noncustodial parents.

Finally, families' social integration was powerfully predicted by the custodial household's family functions, particularly in the later period. Companionship, openness to feedback, and safety—as well as the interaction of conflict with material resources and regularity, and of role boundary flexibility with material resources—were all associated with families' social adjustment. It is striking that the household characteristics do predict family social integration so well and that the noncustodial household characteristics do not play any role. In presenting itself to the social worlds of work, school, and friendship, the custodial household seems, within 18 months, to have genuinely become a "system." The fact that the noncustodial household features are so critical to children's well-being makes clear, though, that it is very much an open system, with powerful ties remaining between children and their fathers, but much weaker ones between mothers and fathers.

NOTES

1. Coding definitions were prepared for each of the various functions, and interview transcripts were coded separately by independent coders, without knowledge of the coding of other variables. Coding definitions and judgments were discussed until raters attained interrater reliability above .85; random spot checks of coding were performed to ensure that reliability was maintained at or above this level.

2. An index combining information about the number of hours worked and the status level of her job; scores for the latter ranged from 1 = no paid employment to 7 = full-time managerial or professional occupations.

3. Coded in terms of mothers' reports of consistency of payment of child support, alimony, and other direct financial support (e.g., payment of rent, tuition, medical expenses, etc.).

4. These three variables were not significantly correlated with each other at either time

(mothers with higher earning capacities sometimes had serious financial difficulties and/or little financial contribution from the father; mothers with lower earning capacities sometimes nevertheless did not experience difficulties obtaining basic necessities). In addition, although mothers' earning capacity was quite stable over time, $r = .79, p < .001$, noncustodial parents' contributions were less stable, $r = .26, p < .05$, and financial difficulties were not stable at all, $r = .14$, ns. Thus, the three variables provided genuinely different information about the custodial household's material resources. They were standardized and combined to create a single index.

5. Different household members' safety concerns were significantly correlated with each other at both times, suggesting that households tended to be experienced similarly by different family members. In addition, reports of safety concerns were quite stable over time (mother and child reports were both correlated, over time, above .40, $p < .001$).

6. Generally, the degree of regularity of routines was fairly stable over time, $r = .39, p < .001$.

7. Scores ranged from 1 (for no joint activities) to 4 (for many specific joint activities) for each reporter for each dyad. Companionship ratings of different household members tended to converge (correlations among reporters averaged about .36, $p < .001$), and they were fairly stable over time (correlations of about .40, $p < .001$).

8. As was described in Chapters 3 and 4, both mothers and children were asked several questions in each interview about the reasons for the separation. Seven categories of reasons occurred in both mother and child responses and could therefore be compared. In addition, coders assessed for each reason whether blame for the separation was attributed to the mother, the father, or both. Parent–child and child–child agreement for reasons and for blame attribution were assessed in terms of the proportion of overall reasons and attributions that were in agreement for each pair. The average agreement across all pairs became the family's overall cohesion score; this score was fairly stable over the period of the study, $r = .31, p < .01$.

9. These scores were not stable over time.

10. Closeness and conflict were uncorrelated at both times, and both were moderately stable over time.

11. These two forms of loyalty strains (child actions and feelings of being caught; direct parent efforts to draw the child into a triangle) were coded on a 3-point scale as rare or absent, present but not frequent, and frequent, according to each custodial household reporter. Aggregate scores were created by summing the two types of loyalty strain scores for each reporter. Each year, about two-thirds of the mothers and one-third of the children reported the presence of some degree of loyalty strain, or triadic relations, involving the target child. Loyalty strains were, as one might expect, somewhat correlated with the reported level of conflict in the mother–father dyad, but these correlations were not high and only significant at Time 2, $r = .18$, ns, and .28, $p < .01$. Over time, loyalty strains were moderately stable, $r = .38, p < .001$.

12. Frequency and regularity were fairly highly correlated at both times (average correlation about .46, $p < .001$). Moreover, frequency and regularity of visits were quite stable over time ($r = .41, p < .001$ for frequency; $r = .29, p < .01$ for regularity). In the 21 mother–father pairs for whom we have both custodial and noncustodial reports on

frequency and regularity of visits, the convergence of the reports was quite high, $r = .63$, $p < .01$, and $.45$, $p < .05$, respectively. See Healy, Malley, and Stewart (1990) for a full account of analyses of the impact of father visitation on children's adjustment.

13. Average correlation between visit frequency and father–child closeness was .40 across years.

14. Tables reporting the details of these analyses are presented in Appendix Tables 10.1 and 10.2.

15. This was accomplished via interaction terms in the regressions.

16. Only significant relationships are displayed in these and subsequent tables; because no relationships with illness were significant for mothers, it is not listed in this table.

17. See Appendix Tables 10.3a and 10.3b for the details of these analyses.

18. See Appendix Tables 10.4a–10.4c for the details of these analyses.

19. See Healy et al. (1990) for a detailed discussion of the relationship between father variables and children's adjustment.

20. A 3-point coding of poor, okay, and good, combined with the proportion of things liked versus disliked about school.

21. Ratings on 4-point scales for up to four school subjects, on the Achenbach CBCL. These ratings were completed on all target children and some siblings.

22. Assessed in terms of a rating of companionate activities from $1 =$ none to $4 =$ frequent. Children's school performance, mothers' work satisfaction, and household members' degree of social involvement with nonhousehold members were all standard-scored and combined into a single index.

23. Details of these analyses are presented in Appendix Table 10.5.

CHAPTER 11

Wise Families, Wise Changes

We have seen in this book that, despite cultural images of divorce as a catastrophe, some families went through this process of family transformation with mothers and children thriving in reorganized households, fathers and children still close, and mothers and fathers in a new kind of relationship to each other, focused on the children's well-being. In some cases, individuals were clearly in better shape after the separation than they had been before; in other cases, individuals and families had simply worked out ways to function and grow that were new and different, but neither better nor worse. There were also some instances in which the separation was still, 18 months later, an overwhelmingly painful event that dominated the daily emotional landscape. One of our primary goals in this project was to see if we could identify factors that enhanced the most positive outcomes for our families. We felt it was important to take stock of what we've found and see if there were things we could advise other families, always recognizing that it is risky to generalize from any one study.

We took stock in three ways: First, we considered folk beliefs about parental separation and whether they were supported by our findings; we also considered what the parents and children we talked to told us *they* would advise others going through separation and divorce; finally, we considered our findings directly and what they might lead us to advise, regardless of folk beliefs or participants' advice. Not surprisingly, we found that many people's advice echoed widespread beliefs in the culture. Perhaps more surprisingly, only some of these beliefs were supported by their own stories. Just going through parental separation, then, does not qualify family members to give good advice about it to others!

This chapter was drafted by Abigail J. Stewart.

We also found, though, that some people gave advice that did accord with our findings, though not necessarily with general cultural beliefs. That advice seemed genuinely "wise," that is, informed by insight, warmth, and compassion for others; practical experience; good judgment; and uncommon sense. The very families that transformed themselves without gratuitous damage or pain in the process had family members who were conscious of the suffering of each other and eager to minimize that suffering, and who recognized the potential for growth and health that parental separation might create for themselves and each other. The ability of these families to continue to meet the needs of family members for individual security and development is testimony to their wisdom.

ABANDONING MYTHS, FINDING THE WISDOM

Both the families that participated in the study and the research team members were well aware of the dominant cultural views about parents and children undergoing separation and divorce. One of our satisfactions in the course of the project, and in looking back at the data, was sifting through these beliefs for the nuggets of wisdom, while abandoning the dusty—and dangerous—myths that too often surround and obscure them.

"Divorce happens because selfish people don't care about their kids' well-being." We found very little evidence to support this view. Even the parents with the least self-control in conflictual situations, and the least success at actually protecting their children, voiced a passionate desire to do the right thing for them. We were struck by the depth of most parents' guilt and anxiety about their children's welfare and the degree to which they had remained in miserable marriages for a long time out of a fear of hurting the children. We also noted that in some cases parents actually decided on separation and divorce only when they were convinced that remaining in the marriage was more harmful to the children (because of violence, economic instability, or uncontainable parental conflict) than leaving it.

Moreover, most parents were anxious about their ability to cope after divorce; for many it took courage and a leap of faith. One woman's advice was:

> "Once you know it's what you want, stick to it. I was really afraid that I wouldn't be able to do it, and that I wouldn't be able to support myself. And it's hard, and I get tired, but it's worth it. I'm not just staying in a situation because I feel trapped anymore."

We do not doubt that there are individual instances of adults who are not sufficiently mindful of their children's well-being and who pursue a private goal at the expense of their family. There probably were individual parents in our sample who did this. But it is inaccurate, cruel, and unjust to the vast majority of parents—including, in many cases, the partners of these selfish individuals—to represent the *average* or *typical* divorcing parents as unconcerned with their children's well-being.

"*Divorce is a catastrophe; it is always bad for children and leaves a trail of misery in its wake.*" Again, we found no evidence to support this folk belief, though many parents we talked with feared that it was true, or were told by friends and relatives that it was, and suffered additional pain because of that fear. We found that parental separation and divorce nearly always felt bad to children, and a very large majority of the children we talked with would have preferred that their parents stay together. This is undeniably true and should not be ignored. It does not mean, though, that parental separation actually should be avoided or that it will have negative effects. Many experiences are unwelcome to some or all children—vaccinations, babysitters, the first day of school, going to camp. But culturally we recognize their real value to children, and we override our children's less informed objections. In the same way, children may (and indeed do) *wish* that their parents would stay together and regret their separation, but they generally lack an understanding of the likely cost to them of depressed, angry, violent, or unhappy parents.

Our evidence and that of many others is that children in fact "adjusted" to parental separation and divorce. Over a relatively short timespan they reported feeling less bad about it, could identify more positive aspects of it, and showed fewer indirect "signs" of distress such as psychological symptoms, behavior problems, or illnesses. Moreover, there is every evidence that parents' well-being was strongly linked with children's, and there is considerable evidence in our data, as well as those of many others, that for many parents the ending of an unhappy marriage initiates a period of personal growth and development, which is good for them and their children.

However, it is clear that for some of the children, even in our sample, parental divorce did *not* end a bad situation. For some, a bad situation simply continued, with parental conflict now taking different forms. For others, parental separation did result in the withdrawal or disengagement of one parent from their lives; for still others, it resulted in increased financial hardship or instability. We do not imagine that every divorce is either neutral or benign in its effects, but the important point is that not every divorce is toxic in its effects. In our view, as a culture our focus should be on supporting positive, and minimizing negative, effects, rather than on condemning the process itself. Ahrons (1995) has called for a recognition that there is such a thing as a "good divorce" and urges us to help couples have them.

Finally, even in the short period we studied, many families had already experienced many new events that were just as important for them as the separation and divorce were. One mother, after an initial anxious period of unemployment, found a vocation and a capacity to support herself she had doubted having. Her transformation in terms of confidence and personal well-being will have a tremendous impact on her children's next 10 years living in her household. In other families, one or the other parent had formed a new and happy relationship and had brought a new adult—sometimes new children—into the family network. These changes, too, will have large and enduring effects on these children's lives. The parental divorce is, in the end, only one event in an individual and family life course that includes *many* significant events; it is a mistake to weight it too heavily.

"Divorce divides one economically viable unit into two, at least one of which is now economically vulnerable." There can be no doubt that divorce has economic consequences; most custodial mothers and their children were worse off financially after the divorce. Moreover, and this is very important, serious material difficulties *were* associated with poorer psychological outcomes for both mothers and the household in the early period. It is also likely that women without the training or capacity for paid employment, and mothers of preschool-age children, faced with the need either to limit their labor force activity or to pay for extensive child care, would have more difficulties than the average woman in our sample. There is reason, then, for concern about the economic vulnerability of mother–child households.

Nevertheless, within this sample of mothers of school-age children, most of whom were employed in the labor force before the separation, mothers generally felt that the gains in personal financial autonomy after the separation offset the losses in financial resources. And the negative psychological impact of fewer material resources was, for the sample as a whole, absent by the time of the follow-up (though, of course, this was not necessarily true for particularly strapped individual households). In short, parental separation did destabilize the families economically, and both mothers and children were negatively affected. Mothers did, however, see advantages as well as disadvantages in their postseparation financial situation, and most adapted fairly quickly. While we have a collective social responsibility to mitigate the negative economic impact of divorce for women and children, our evidence does not suggest that the economic implications of divorce—*by themselves*—should serve as a major deterrent to it.

"When there is a separation or divorce, children's mothers should stay at home (shouldn't work outside the home) so as to be available to their children." We found no evidence to support this idea, at least in this sample of mothers with at least one school-age child. In fact, we found that working outside the home was generally beneficial to the mothers' well-being (which in turn was beneficial to the children's). Even so, for women who had not worked outside

the home before the separation, or who viewed their family and work responsibilities as in conflict, increased labor force activity was *not* beneficial.

In itself, having a mother who was employed full-time outside the home was, if anything, associated with children's better adjustment, but mostly it had little impact. Some types of children—for example, those with well-developed interpersonal judgment—actually found it more difficult to have a mother at home full-time, while those with lesser skills found it easier.

It seems clear, then, that "one size" of maternal employment does not fit all mothers or all children. Although we cannot prescribe the right amount of employment outside the home in all cases, we do note two important points. First, most of the mothers in our study had no financial alternative to employment; they were providing financially for their children by working, and they simply had to do it. Second, working—for pay or on some other basis—felt to many women like a therapeutic, supportive, or helpful activity. One mother said:

> "I think it would be just atrocious to have a life in which it was just you and the children, getting divorced and living in your house. You need something that's yours, in which you're interacting with other adults—whether that's a full-time job, a part-time job, going to school—you need the opportunity to have a life for yourself."

"If a divorce takes place, everything else should stay the same." We found little or no evidence that other kinds of simultaneous changes—moves, changes of schools, and so forth—were good or bad in their effects during this period. There's no doubt that nearly all the parents *believed* that change would be bad for their kids. For example, one mother said she would advise "trying to keep everything as much the same as possible—not moving, not changing schools, basically keeping as much of the same routine as possible." A noncustodial father had a similar view:

> "I think one thing that has helped the most with the kids is the relative sameness of everything else in their lives, i.e., same house, same school, same friends, same general activities. So the only thing that changed was that I wasn't there anymore every day."

Despite parents' confidence that sameness was helpful, and that change would be problematic, we found no evidence to support this. The children from the relatively small number of families that did make major changes were no better or worse off than the children from the much larger group of families that avoided changes. This is particularly striking because we did find that children (and their mothers) did not do well in the postseparation period if they did not feel safe and secure. Presumably the reason people imagine that change is problematic during this period is that they expect it to threaten children's sense of stability and security, but by itself change doesn't seem to have that effect.

It is certainly possible that, as most families *did* avoid change, the families that made changes were really different from the others in some important way from those that didn't. In particular, these may have been families in which changes were really desired by family members for reasons unconnected to the divorce. For example, Mary Maxwell (introduced in Chapter 1) moved her children away from an isolated community into a more active neighborhood. Perhaps they all viewed that as a change that improved their lives. The point, then, may be that changes should be considered in light of their relative capacity to improve the family's situation or to threaten family members' sense of security, *rather* than as uniformly dangerous and problematic.

"Conflict between parents is always bad for children." This belief was probably the one that was best supported by our data, as by many other studies. It is clear that parental conflict *was* mostly bad for children, and that an important goal for separating and divorcing parents should be to minimize or contain the conflict. Some parents told us they thought that "if you think your ex is a jerk, he probably is, and it's better for your children to know it." Although some parents believed that this was "honest," or "open," we did not find evidence that this kind of openness or honesty was in fact helpful, or even neutral, for children. Parental conflict when parents are married is painful and destructive to children; getting away from that conflict is one of the potential benefits of divorce. One wise 10-year-old offered this advice to other children about parental divorce:

> "I'd tell them that it isn't so bad. It's a good influence 'cause if they stayed together for a few years and they were arguing it'd be a real bad influence on you. That's exactly what I'd tell them."

Parental conflict was especially harmful under certain circumstances: when children were young (under 9 in our sample) and when the conflict was violent and/or persistent over time. Even more powerfully, we found that being directly brought into parental conflict—creating loyalty strains—was *the single most consistent predictor of worse adjustment for children.* One wise father said:

> "I've seen some parents through my life that, as soon as they get the kid, they start playing '20 questions.' I would never do that. But I've seen children who have gone through that. And the minute the child is dropped off [by the other parent] they call up and they start yelling at

their old wife or husband. It's ridiculous. When they are out of the house, forget it; as long as the child is being well taken care of, that's your only concern."

Parental conflict was also associated with poorer well-being for mothers, *particularly* if the conflict revolved around issues having to do with the children (custody, visitation, etc.). Both mothers and children, though, were not so negatively affected by parental conflict once the divorce had become final. It seems clear that part of the toxicity of conflict comes from the fear that it signals instability or uncertainty about everyday life. When it loses that "signal" value, it loses some of its harmful effect. This may account for the fact that the only family members who did not seem harmed by parental conflict were the fathers; perhaps conflict rarely or never seemed to them to carry with it a risk to everyday life.

"In the course of divorce, parental conflict is inevitable." At the time of the separation, parents' general emotional orientation toward proactivity and getting their needs met may increase the chances that divorcing couples will be aware of conflicting needs and goals. However, even if conflict in the sense of disagreement, or divergent perspectives, is inevitable in the course of divorce, we found *no* evidence that conflict in the sense of arguing and fighting was inevitable. Instead, we found that some families experienced little or no fighting once the decision to separate was made; in others, conflict was contained and children were separated from it. (It should be noted that some couples who did not fight created different problems for their children—e.g., mystification about why the divorce was happening. But much more typically, "not fighting" was associated with other good things, like being able to work together to benefit the children.)

The couples who contained their conflict tended to be the ones who focused on creating a new, coparenting relationship and who let go of the frustration, anger, or disappointment that may have been connected with their failed marriage. One father described it to us this way:

"The thing is the talking. The rational talking where the child is involved, where you're involved, and your [ex-]wife is involved. The main interest should be the child. It is beautiful. I didn't think I could do this, and she didn't think she could do it, but we found out that it helps her, it helps me, and it helps the child. And if this keeps up, the child will be brought up well."

For this family it was *work* to contain the conflict and create a new, "rational" coparenting relationship. But it was work that this father felt was paying off for all of them.

"*Because parental divorce is a change—and an unwanted one for children—it is very important to maintain regular routines for them.*" This is another case where it seems to us that the truth is more complicated than folk beliefs; and where folk beliefs can in fact create problems for struggling parents. In families with at least one school-age child, regular routines were not, overall, of much importance. However, it *did* seem that regular routines in the household were helpful when interpersonal conflict among household members were high. Our guess is that the stability and predictability of the routines offset some of the anxiety about security that conflict generated. However, when conflict was low, regular routines actually were associated with poorer outcomes, probably because that regularity was not fulfilling a real need (as in the case of the conflictual families), but was motivated by some kind of rigidity for its own sake.

Regularity of children's visitation with their noncustodial fathers was *also* not always good, probably for similar reasons. When parental conflict was high, more regular visits were associated with worse outcomes—probably because the regular visits were associated with regular fights. More irregular visitation may be more spontaneous, may therefore help minimize conflict in these families, and thus may be more helpful to children.

Similarly, regular visits with their fathers were associated with good outcomes for boys, especially younger ones, but not for girls, especially older ones. It may well be that the security associated with a regular pattern of visitation was particularly reassuring to younger boys, but felt particularly confining to older girls, who may more often have had interests they did not share with their fathers and even some discomfort about managing their relationship with him without an adult woman present. The evidence that male children were more often "fought over" than females suggests another, more disturbing, possibility. Perhaps girls did worse with more contact with their fathers because they felt their fathers' did not value or appreciate them (while boys felt highly prized). Recall that Anita Anderson (Chapter 1) missed her difficult mother because "it's hard living in a house with all boys." She felt that her father had much more in common with her brother: "I'm not a boy, so there's nothing he can relate to." Even if noncustodial fathers do value and appreciate their daughters as much as their sons, it's possible that they share fewer interests with them and are more uncertain about how to talk with them. Their discomfort and awkwardness could feel like rejection to their anxious daughters.

We did find that having an emotionally *close* relationship with their father *was* uniformly good for children (suggesting that both boys and girls benefit from closeness, but that regularity and frequency may not always signal it). The point, then, is that it is the *relationship* that matters; when that relationship is tricky, it may be important for there to be room for space and spontaneity.

"It is very important for children to maintain close ties with the noncusto-
dial parent (in our case usually the father) after parental divorce." On the whole
this *was* true, but the point is the *quality of the relationship*, not the more
practical features of it. However, the frequency and regularity of father visitation showed much more complex patterns. For boys and younger children
contact itself was associated with good outcomes, but for girls and older children it was actually problematic. As we have seen, issues of developmental
autonomy, gender, and loyalty pressures may be at stake in these findings, but
the most important point is that it is *not* reasonable to prescribe any particular pattern of contact for children and their noncustodial parents. What *is*
reasonable is to try to enhance the quality and closeness of their relationship,
however frequently or regularly they see each other.

It was, by the way, equally true that a good, close relationship between
the custodial mother and her children was critical to her children's and her
own well-being; that relationship also cannot be taken for granted. One
mother's advice to others pointed this out:

"The best advice would be just to reinforce the love that you have for
your children. Try to get closer to them. Just let them know that you're
there and that you're willing to listen and you understand what's happening and just offer to help them."

"After a parental separation or divorce, it's important for the single parent to
establish and maintain firm authority over the household." Firm role boundaries
between mothers and children were not associated, in general, with good *or*
bad outcomes for children. But they were associated with *worse* outcomes for
mothers themselves. The complexity of the issues involved in single-parent
families' role structure was captured in one mother's advice to others:

"Try to emphasize the positive. Say, 'Life is an adventure and it's a new
challenge and we're all going to meet this one together.' I think before,
when you're married, I think you and your husband meet the adventure
together and the children aren't pulled into it as much. I think also that
[after a separation] they should have more input into the decision making. The final decision has to be yours, but they need to be a little more
part of it, because in a sense as a group, you need to interact more, because you don't have an interaction partner. But you also have to be very
careful to be sure that you don't use your children in an adult's capacity."

What this mother makes abundantly clear is that the single parent is in a *dif-*
ferent relationship with her children than is the married parent, and that she
needs to calibrate the firmness of the boundaries between adult and children
in new and flexible ways.

The importance of flexibility was underscored in other findings. For example, it was clear that when family members of different developmental stages and positions in the household shared a perspective on the divorce, this was not a good thing either for individual family members or for the family's overall social integration. We suspect that having a cohesive viewpoint about the divorce across generations may be the result of particularly unpleasant family situations, or of pressure toward conformity, which is confining in much the same way as unnecessarily rigid role boundaries.

Finally, we found that being in a family in which it was possible openly to express critical views was very good for children. One mother, who seemed particularly attuned to the reasons this might be important for children, said:

"Keep talking to them. Let them talk. Don't be afraid of them hurting you, don't be afraid—let them say it. Don't think of yourself and say, 'I don't want to hear your father's name mentioned.' Try not to let your own hurt cut them off and let them have no way to express it. . . . If you're wrong, admit your mistakes. And try to explain why you [made] them, and that you wouldn't do that again, but calling the shots the way they are, you would probably do the same thing again."

She recommended a kind of freedom from defensiveness and vulnerability that may be difficult for a divorcing parent to muster, but it is not difficult to imagine how positive that stance would be for her children. Rigid role boundaries, a shared view of an event that is inherently asymmetrical in its effects, and being closed to critical feedback are all features of postseparation families that would tend to inhibit and constrain children from articulating their own feelings and perspective, and thereby coming to terms with them.

"Divorce is always hardest on boys and young children." We found virtually no evidence to support these ideas, within the age range of our sample (school-age children). Boys and girls showed somewhat different kinds of "symptoms"; boys were more likely to be seen as having behavior problems, whereas girls had more physical symptoms and reported more emotional distress. But these gender differences are characteristic of many samples of boys and girls, not just those with divorcing parents.

Similarly, we found no sign that younger (or older) children were worse off, but there was some evidence that older children's psychological adjustment, and younger children's physical adjustment, improved more quickly over the period we studied. This may indicate that children of different ages are resilient in different ways, but it does not suggest that they differ in their overall resilience. The one indication of younger children's greater vulnerability lies in the larger impact of parental conflict on them. There is no reason to think that impact is a function of the parental divorce; parental conflict in the *absence* of divorce may also be more destructive for younger children (see, e.g., Block, Block, & Morrison, 1981).

Overall, conventional "wisdom" about divorce isn't very wise, in our view. Moreover, it ignores some aspects of divorce that are, according to our findings, very important.

IMPLICATIONS OF CONSIDERING PARENTAL SEPARATION A PROCESS

Thinking of parental separation as an event that is part of a process of family transformation highlights several aspects of parental separation that do turn out to matter. First, we are forced to take account of the past—a painful, complicated story of unhappiness (and sometimes confinement, violence, and pathology) in a marriage. Once we do that, it is much more difficult simply to recommend that people avoid separation and divorce.

Second, we are forced to take account of the future—to notice that pain diminishes and symptoms of distress subside, even over 1 year. Moreover, there are signs of new growth and development, perhaps especially for women. Thus, considering parental separation a process helps refocus our attention on divorce as providing families with an opportunity to change negative or destructive features of their lives and to replace them with more positive, growth-promoting ones.

Finally, thinking of parental separation as a process reminds us that different things matter at different times. We found this to be especially true for the adults. New single parents needed to focus on concrete tasks in the early period, and they and their children were helped if the divorce was settled quickly. As one mother put it:

> "I think that doing things very quickly was very good for everybody because it avoided long, drawn-out hassles and that, I think, is definitely worth doing.
>
> On a practical side, try to do in advance some of the things I did. I had two gasoline credit cards in my name. I applied for two others and got them before [my ex-husband] moved out so that at least I was able to charge gasoline on my own card . . . I didn't have a Mastercard or a Visa card and that would have been easier if I had been able to apply in advance for that."

It seems clear that concrete, practical issues must be addressed early and quickly if parents are to move on to other matters.

At the same time, we found that emotional support, which didn't appear to be important early on, turned out to matter over time and at the time of the follow-up. This same mother said, even in the first interview, "I also think some of the things that helped me are I talked to some other women who were divorced or separated." In the follow-up interview she was even more convinced: "Find somebody else who's in the same situation that you're in . . . so you have someone to talk to who has been there." Many other mothers stressed the importance of social support, though not always from people in the same situation. One mother said:

> "It's important to have someone that you can talk to, whether it be a social worker or counselor or a minister or your mother or just a good friend. Just don't feel defeated by it. You can make it."

Our study ends very much in the middle of these families' stories. Their lives have gone on to include other tasks, other events, other challenges. By seeing the divorce as part of a process, we begin to see it within a stream of events of greater and lesser importance and to weigh it accordingly.

IMPLICATIONS OF CONSIDERING PARENTAL DIVORCE A SYSTEM EVENT

We are struck by the value of viewing parental divorce as an event that affects a family *system*, not merely a collection of individuals. By doing so, we are immediately attuned to the fact that this event affects different parts of the system differently. We found that parents and children were profoundly "out of synch" at the point of parental separation—with parents at the end of a long process of coming to terms with an increasingly untenable personal relationship, and children at the beginning of a process of coming to terms with the dissolution of a familiar household structure. Similarly, parents were, at the time of the separation, ready to embrace a proactive stance toward the world while children instead adopted a reactive, receptive stance. We suspect that children's well-being would be enhanced if parents understood the difference in their stances in very concrete terms.

Because parental separation faces children with upsetting, new information, they have certain needs that are different from their parents; for example, they need to understand what is, and what is not, implied by parental separation, something parents have usually long since worked out for themselves. One mother demonstrated her awareness of her children's need for explanations in her advice to "share everything, or almost everything, with your children." She said, "Share with them, don't shut them out because they're scared." One of the noncustodial fathers mentioned in the course of his advice that

"I think being able to show them immediately where I was going to live probably allayed a lot of fears that they might have had. You know, it's 10 minutes away from where they live, and so on. And having them come to spend a night or two in the new place fairly quickly after I moved in was probably good. And, I guess, answering their questions honestly. 'Where are you going to live? Are you going to get married?'"

Some parents are so preoccupied with their own concerns, and so unaware that their children's concerns are very different, that they may not address these early needs for reassurance so directly and so completely. But our evidence shows that freedom from anxiety and uncertainty is one of the most important factors in children's adjustment.

We have also pointed out that parental conflict is probably such a potent factor in children's adjustment primarily because of the way it raises anxiety about how stable or permanent postseparation arrangements really are. It may also be that children's general passive receptivity at this time amplifies the impact of strong external stimuli. If parents understood that parental conflict during this early period makes children anxious and fearful about their lives (but apparently doesn't once the divorce is settled), perhaps they could more effectively shield them from it, or at least address the anxiety it generates. Similarly, conflict that directly affects children, or that traps them in loyalty strains, can be understood as especially likely to be anxiety provoking, and therefore especially to be avoided.

A second major implication of taking a systems view is that it leads us both to define the system carefully and to notice that it is a system embedded in a set of relationships with other systems. The postseparation family must be defined not in terms of a single household, but in terms of two loosely connected households. Once we take this seriously, we can discover—as we did in this study—that features of the noncustodial household have tremendous impact on children's well-being, but not on mothers' and not on the custodial households' as a whole. These findings make perfect sense when we recognize that, indeed, it is children who create the permeability of the boundary between the two households. It is inevitable, then, that they will be influenced by what goes on on both sides of that boundary in a way that neither parent will be. If parents recognize the great importance of ex-spouses' households for their children, despite the (welcome) irrelevance for parents, they may be more able to accept, even facilitate, their ex-spouses as coparents. As a culture, we do not generally encourage and support the creation of healthy "binuclear" households. Full recognition of this family form might lead friends and family, as well as helping professionals, to develop methods for supporting and encouraging the development of healthy coparenting relationships to replace unsatisfactory marriages.

At the same time, once we recognize the family as a system, we also must attend to the other systems with which it is connected. We have seen how important mothers' and children's social ties—at work and school, and with friends and extended families—are to their postseparation well-being. And we have seen that the noncustodial household factors were *not* important predictors of the custodial household's social integration or the mothers' well-being. Thus, a system view helps us to recognize both areas that are, in fact, *not* key points for intervention, as well as the wider context in which the family operates. The need to identify how divorcing families could get more support (and less stress and pain) from related systems like work, school, and neighborhoods is underscored by a systems perspective and our findings.

Similarly, viewing parental separation from a systems perspective allows us to accept the single-parent household as a new system with its own integrity and nature, *different* from a two-parent system. We have seen that single-parent families may be especially challenged in providing children (and mothers) with a sense of safety and security, perhaps especially because their material resources are likely to be limited and parental conflict high. Single-parent households may be better served than two-parent ones by careful construction of participatory household decision-making structures, rather than firm role boundaries. And single parents may need to be encouraged to be flexible and creative in creating new family routines and procedures that suit their households. Finally, single-parent families need to be encouraged not to focus solely inward, but to turn their attention to the supports available outside the household system.

A systems perspective on the divorcing family helps us notice some ways in which gender operates at a systems level in these families. Some families were rigidly gender differentiated before the separation. For some women that was a source of tension, which led them to seek escape from a confining set of expectations. This may account for the fact that more women initiate divorces (in our sample and most others) and more women than men in our sample reported positive growth after the separation. For some of the men in our study, the wife's effort to change the gender structure of the household was indeed a factor in their own dissatisfaction with the marriage; for others, it was simply mystifying. In addition, the new, postseparation gender structure in most of our families' lives (mother-headed custodial households and father-headed noncustodial ones) seemed to have important implications. A systems perspective helps focus attention on the gender system as it is reflected in families before and after separation.

Finally, a systems perspective helps us identify interconnections where they exist. Recognizing the interconnectedness of the individuals, dyads, and triads in the family can be an important source of both empowerment and relief from guilt. For example, we have seen that the quality of the mother–child relationship is related to both mothers' and children's well-being. We have also seen that it is related to father–child conflict and to extrafamily support of the mother. Thus, individuals, dyads, and systems are all interconnected. What that suggests is that if we change any one of these elements, we can influence them all. If we see a mother and child who have a bad relationship, both of whom are showing symptoms of poor adjustment, we can reasonably expect that an improvement in extrafamilial support to the mother or a diminution of parental conflict (or both) would lead to a better relationship *and* better adjustment of both. Interconnectedness, then, can lead us to a wider range of potentially relevant solutions to problems.

At the same time, adoption of a systems perspective can lead us away from worrying about aspects of situations we cannot change and free us from guilt about them. Thus, for example, we have found that parental conflict is destructive to children and should be curbed. What if a parent is divorcing a person who is high in power motivation and low in responsibility, and who therefore is likely to engage in conflict, regardless of his/her partner's responses? Can the parent reasonably expect to lower the partner's power motivation or increase their partner's responsibility? Of course not. But a systems perspective reminds us that *other* factors also shape adjustment, and one of them is regularity of visitation. When the noncustodial parent is particularly explosive, perhaps adopting a more flexible visitation schedule would help contain the conflict. Taking a systems perspective can help us ignore or forgive the things that cannot be changed because it encourages us to identify *other* things that *can* be changed. Alternatively, it may lead us to identify the *aspect* of something that is problematic so we can change that. For example, our data suggest that sophisticated social-cognitive abilities can jeopardize children's adjustment if their mothers are not employed full-time. Obviously we can't *lower* children's social cognitive abilities—and we probably wouldn't want to! But we can think about *why* social-cognitive abilities have a negative effect (probably because they increase children's empathy-based anxiety about her well-being) and take steps to mitigate that effect indirectly (for example, the mother could avoid displaying her negative feelings to the child or could encourage the child's independent activities outside the home). Recognizing that the family is a system, and that every individual, dyad, and triad is a subsystem of it, can help parents and helping professionals to identify points of intervention that might work *because* of the interconnectedness of all of the elements of it.

FAMILY TRANSFORMATIONS

Families change their size and shape throughout their histories. They add new members when children are born or adopted. They lose a member when someone dies. Their boundaries are stretched when members go away to school or "grow up and leave home." But throughout those changes we recognize them still as families, and as whole ones at that. We never think a home in which a parent has died is "broken"; it has faced a painful loss, but the family is recognized as enduring.

In our judgment, when parents separate and divorce, it is no less true that a family endures—with a new shape (see Weiss, 1975, for a related argument). As a culture we have been willing to recognize some family changes as acceptable, or uncontrollable; but we have resisted treating parental separation and divorce as either acceptable or uncontrollable. Despite that fact, our data suggest that even without cultural support for it, many families find healthy ways to make the transition from a one-household to a two-household family. We hope for the day when this particular family transformation will be treated, as now, as a painful last resort for the unhappily married, but at the same time as a potentially growth-promoting opportunity. When that day comes more families may be able to make use of that opportunity.

We note, too, that family events rarely define and label individuals forever. We don't refer to children whose fathers were killed in wars as "children of death." Although we recognize the "empty nest" as a phenomenon, we rarely refer to parents who occupy those nests by name. No family event fully defines any individual family member; how could it, when all families take many shapes over time, with none of them lasting very long? Parental separation and divorce are part of an important process of family transformation—one we obviously thought deserved study! But it is only *one* process in a family history that extends forward and backward in time and includes many other significant events. We must respect, but not overestimate, its role in family members' lives.

APPENDIX TABLES

APPENDIX TABLE 3.1. Mothers' Adjustment over Time

	Average score at:		
Measure ($n = 96$)	Time 1	Time 2	Significance of change
Total mood disturbance[a]	45.28	28.68	*p* < .001
Anger–hostility	15.05	9.69	*p* < .001
Confusion–bewilderment	9.03	6.32	*p* < .001
Depression–dejection	13.75	9.98	*p* < .01
Tension–anxiety	13.75	10.53	*p* < .001
Fatigue–inertia	9.85	8.22	*p* < .01
Vigor–activity	15.92	16.08	
Self-esteem[b]	32.25	32.71	ns
Life satisfaction[c]	2.83	3.03	*p* < .05
Psychological symptoms[d]	35.62	33.00	*p* < .001
Psychological anxiety	11.45	10.67	*p* < .001
Illness	7.39	6.99	*p* < .10
Immobilization	8.71	7.87	*p* < .001

[a]Based on the six subscales of the POMS (McNair et al., 1971)
[b]Based on Rosenberg's (1965) measure of self-esteem.
[c]One 4-point item, ranging from 1 = not very satisfied to 4 = completely satisfied.
[d]Overall scale and subscales from measure of stress symptoms used by Gurin et al. (1960) and Veroff et al. (1981).

APPENDIX TABLE 3.2. Fathers' Adjustment over Time

	Average score at:		
Measure ($n = 34$)	Time 1	Time 2	Significance of change
Total mood disturbance[a]	41.97	20.19	*p* < .001
Anger–hostility	11.83	6.60	*p* < .01
Confusion–bewilderment	9.03	6.54	*p* < .01
Depression–dejection	14.49	8.68	*p* < .01
Tension–anxiety	13.24	8.57	*p* < .01
Fatigue–inertia	8.24	6.32	ns
Vigor–activity	15.08	15.68	ns
Self-esteem[b]	33.09	34.46	ns
Life satisfaction[c]	2.39	3.00	*p* < .05
Psychological symptoms[d]	31.13	29.00	ns
Psychological anxiety	9.79	9.21	*p* < .05
Illness	6.32	6.18	ns
Immobilization	7.51	7.59	ns

[a]Based on the six subscales of the POMS (McNair et al., 1971)
[b]Based on Rosenberg's (1965) measure of self-esteem.
[c]One 4-point item, ranging from 1 = not very satisfies to 4 = completely satisfied.
[d]Overall scale and subscales from measure of stress symptoms used by Gurin et al. (1960) and Veroff et al. (1981).

APPENDIX TABLE 4.1. Children's Adjustment over Time

Measure ($n = 98$)	Average score at:		Significance of change
	Time 1	Time 2	
Psychological adjustment[a]	0.617	0.680	$p < .05$
Illness[b]	1.142	1.123	ns
Behavior problems (mother-reported)[c]	35.974	30.147	$p < .05$
Behavior problems (teacher-reported)[d]	10.556	7.303	$p < .05$

Note. See Appendix Table 6.2 for breakdown by age an gender.
[a]Self-report index, including Perceived Competence Scale (Harter, 1982), adaptation of Twenty Symptoms (Veroff et al. 1981), and divorce-related feelings (see Chapter 2).
[b]Mother reports of children's illnesses in previous 3 months.
[c]Mother reports on the CBCL (see Achenbach, 1978).
[d]Teacher reports on the CBCL (Edelbrock & Achenbach, 1984).

APPENDIX TABLE 5.1. Correlations between Time 1 Predictor Variables and Mothers' Adjustment, Time 1 and Time 2

	Time 1		Time 2	
	Psychological adjustment ($n = 121$)[a]	Illness ($n = 121$)[a]	Psychological adjustment ($n = 103$)[a]	Illness ($n = 103$)[a]
Support for day-to-day demands, Time 1				
Preseparation paid employment				
Total sample	.19*	−.20	.07	−.26*
Preschool children in family ($n = 47$)[a]	.32*	−.42*	.11	−.37*
Adolescent children in family ($n = 34$)[a]	.46*	−.06	.31	−.31
Higher job status				
Total sample	.26*	−.13	.07	−.24*
High interparent conflict ($n = 59$)[a]	.45**	−.20	.34*	−.35*
Worsened financial situation				
Total sample	−.19	.03	−.19	.12
Preschool children in family ($n = 47$)[a]	−.38*	.26	−.24	.28
Practical help				
Total sample	.26**	−.28**	.17	−.21*
Mother employed full-time ($n = 66$)[a]	.29*	−.31*	.16	−.21
High legal conflict ($n = 62$)[a]	.31*	−.36*	.17	−.25
Support for psychological growth, Time 1				
Emotional support				
Total sample	.13	−.04	.21*	−.17
Mother not employed full-time ($n = 48$)	.24	−.24	.34*	−.38*
Affiliation motivation				
Total sample	−.06	.08	.14	−.09
Conflict with ex-spouse				
Total sample	.10	.04	−.16	.23*
Power motivation				
Total sample	−.18	.06	−.31**	.26*

[a]n's vary from this maximum depending upon availability of data.
*$p < .05$; **$p < .01$.

APPENDIX TABLE 5.2. Correlations between Time 2 Predictor Variables and Mothers' Adjustment, Time 2

	Psychological adjustment $(n = 103)^a$	Illness $(n = 103)^a$
Support for day-to-day demands		
Paid employment		
Total sample	.01	−.08
Higher job status		
Total sample	.03	−.00
High legal conflict $(n = 42)^a$	.25	−.38*
Work–family conflict		
Total sample	−.45***	.14
Preschool children in family $(n = 29)^a$	−.56**	.08
Divorce not settled $(n = 37)^a$	−.58***	.06
Practical help		
Total sample	−.11	−.02
Support for psychological growth		
Emotional support		
Total sample	.15	−.09
Affiliation motivation		
Total sample	−.05	.07
Dating		
Total sample	.24*	−.25*
Conflict with ex-spouse		
Total sample	−.18	.16
Power motivation		
Total sample	−.23*	.23*

*$p < .05$; **$p < .01$; ***$p < .001$.
$^a n$'s vary from this maximum depending upon availability of data.

APPENDIX TABLE 5.3. Correlations between Predictor Variables and Fathers' Adjustment, Time 1 and Time 2

	Time 1		Time 2	
	Psychological adjustment $(n = 49)^a$	Illness $(n = 49)^a$	Psychological adjustment $(n = 34)^a$	Illness $(n = 34)^a$
Support for day-to-day demands				
Job status, Time 1	−.16	−.29	−.27†	−.23
Support for psychological growth				
Emotional support, Time 1	−.06	.45*	.06	.47*
Emotional support, Time 2	—	—	.20	.40†
Dating, Time 2	—	—	.42†	−.06
Affiliation motivation, Time 1	−.60**	.12	−.28	.28
Affiliation motivation, Time 2	—	—	−.37†	.15

†$p < .10$; *$p < .05$; **$p < .01$.
$^a n$'s vary from this maximum depending upon availability of data.

APPENDIX TABLE 6.1. Pearson Correlations between Child
Adjustment Measures

	Psychological adjustment $(n = 95)^a$	Illness $(n = 105)^a$	Behavior problems (mother-rated) $(n = 104)^a$	Behavior problems (teacher-rated) $(n = 73)^a$
Psychological adjustment		−.22*	−.38***	−.23*
Illness	.01		.11	.17
Behavior problems (mother-rated)	−.22*	.08		.36**
Behavior problems (teacher-rated)	−.16	−.10	.41***	

Note. Correlations above the diagonal refer to within-Time 1 relationships; correlations below the diagonal refer to within-Time 2 relationships.

^{a}n's vary from this maximum depending upon availability of data.

*$p < .05$; **$p < .025$; ***$p < .001$.

APPENDIX TABLE 6.2. Age × Sex × Time Means for Child Adjustment
Measures

	Psychological adjustment	Illness	Behavior problems (mother-rated)	Behavior problems (teacher-rated)
Time 1				
Older boys $(n = 25)^a$	0.59	1.12	37.52	14.00
Older girls $(n = 22)^a$	0.63	1.15	32.53	6.00
Younger boys $(n = 24)^a$	0.65	1.10	41.54	17.00
Younger girls $(n = 27)^a$	0.60	1.20	32.30	5.22
Time 2				
Older boys	0.69	1.10	33.88	11.80
Older girls	0.72	1.22	26.41	6.90
Younger boys	0.68	1.07	33.21	6.07
Younger girls	0.64	1.10	27.09	4.44

^{a}n's vary from this maximum depending upon availability of data.

APPENDIX TABLE 6.2a. Age × Sex × Time Repeated-Measures Analysis of Variance for Psychological Adjustment Measure

Source	SS	df	MS	F
Sex	.01	1	.01	0.07
Age	.01	1	.01	0.23
Sex × Age	.07	1	.07	1.67
Error	3.83	91	.04	
Time	.19	1	.19	16.97***
Sex × Time	.00	1	.00	0.02
Age × Time	.05	1	.05	4.84*
Sex × Age × Time	.00	1	.00	0.20
Error	1.01	91	.01	
Total	5.17	189	.03	

$*p < .05; ***p < .001.$

APPENDIX TABLE 6.2b. Age × Sex × Time Repeated-Measures Analysis of Variance for Illness Measure

Source	SS	df	MS	F
Sex	.09	1	.19	5.10*
Age	.04	1	.04	1.00
Sex × Age	.00	1	.00	0.07
Error	3.16	85	.04	
Time	.02	1	.02	0.82
Sex × Time	.00	1	.00	0.10
Age × Time	.09	1	.09	4.79*
Sex × Age × Time	.07	1	.07	3.68†
Error	1.61	85	.02	
Total	5.18	177	.03	

$†p < .10; *p < .05.$

APPENDIX TABLE 6.2c. Age × Sex × Time Repeated-Measures Analysis of Variance for Mother-Rated Behavior Problems Measures

Source	SS	df	MS	F
Sex	2,103.12	1	2103.12	2.55
Age	39.25	1	39.25	0.05
Sex × Age	22.86	1	22.86	0.03
Error	70,113.63	85	824.87	
Time	1,476.56	1	1,476.56	11.28***
Sex × Time	1.11	1	1.11	0.01
Age × Time	39.10	1	39.10	0.03
Sex × Age × Time	85.04	1	85.04	0.65
Error	11,124.63	85	130.88	
Total	85,004.63	177	480.25	

***$p < .001$.

APPENDIX TABLE 6.2d. Age × Sex × Time Repeated-Measures Analysis of Variance for Teacher-Rated Behavior Problems Measures

Source	SS	df	MS	F
Sex	915.47	1	915.47	7.07*
Age	47.12	1	47.12	0.36
Sex × Age	0.33	1	0.33	0.00
Error	5,179.72	40	129.49	
Time	224.06	1	224.06	5.20*
Sex × Time	232.56	1	232.56	5.40*
Age × Time	143.46	1	143.46	3.33†
Sex × Age × Time	65.89	1	65.89	1.53
Error	1,723.49	40	43.09	
Total	8,532.08	87	98.07	

†$p < .10$; *$p < .05$.

APPENDIX TABLE 6.3. Relationships between Child Adjustment and
Postseparation Household Situation, Time 1

Household situation	Psychological adjustment ($n = 120$)	Illness ($n = 105$)	Behavior problems (mother-rated) ($n = 104$)	Behavior problems (teacher-rated) ($n = 73$)
Mother employed[a]	.03	−.05	−.24*	−.05
Recent changes[b]	.02	.09	.01	.01
Parental conflict[c]	−.11	.12	.21*	.25*

[a]High score = mother employed full-time.
[b]High score = higher number of recent changes.
[c]High score = more parental conflict.
*$p < .05$.

APPENDIX TABLE 6.4. Relationships between Peer Support Measures
and Adjustment

Peer support measure	Psychological adjustment ($n = 115$)[a]	Illness ($n = 103$)[a]	Behavior problems (mother-rated) ($n = 102$)[a]	Behavior problems (teacher-rated) ($n = 70$)[a]
Activities with friends	.06	.06	.01	−.09
Activities with siblings	.02	.15	−.02	−.16

[a]n's vary from this maximum due to missing data.

APPENDIX TABLE 6.5. Relationships between Child Adjustment and
Individual Characteristics

	Psychological adjustment ($n = 120$)[a]	Illness ($n = 105$)[a]	Behavior problems (mother-rated) ($n = 104$)[a]	Behavior problems (teacher-rated) ($n = 73$)[a]
Within Time 1				
Perspective taking	.01	−.08	−.02	−.11
Person concepts	.01	−.22*	−.18	−.01
Self-consciousness	−.43***	.02	.20*	.13
Internal locus of control	−.09	.00	−.11	−.28*
Within Time 2				
Perspective taking	.03	.02	.20	.01
Person concepts	.01	.03	.11	.14
Self-consciousness	−.27*	.13	.15	.11
Internal locus of control	−.01	.03	−.20	−.09

[a]n's vary from this maximum depending upon availability of data.
*$p < .05$; ***$p < .001$.

APPENDIX TABLE 6.6. Multiple Regressions: Significance of Interaction Terms in Analyses Involving Parental Conflict and Ways of Understanding and Peer Support Variables Predicting Adjustment for Boys and Girls Combined

	Time 1 measures Time 1 adjustment $(n = 120)^a$		Time 1 measures Time 2 adjustment $(n = 120)^a$		Time 2 measures Time 2 adjustment $(n = 100)^a$	
	p^b	R^c	p^b	R^c	p^b	R^c
Psychological adjustment						
Perspective taking	**	.29*	*	.27†		
Person concepts						
Self-consciousness						
Internal locus of control	**	.29*	**	.32*		
Friend activities			*	.31*		
Sibling activities						
Illness						
Perspective taking						
Person concepts						
Self-consciousness						
Internal locus of control	*	.23				
Friend activities						
Sibling activities	**	.33**				
Behavior problems (mother-rated)						
Perspective taking						
Person concepts						
Self-consciousness					†	.30*
Internal locus of control	*	.34**				
Friend activities						
Sibling activities						
Behavior problems (teacher-rated)						
Perspective taking						
Person concepts						
Self-consciousness						
Internal locus of control	***	.58***				
Friend activities	*	.37*				
Sibling activities						

Note. Interpretations of interaction effects are provided in the text.
[a]n's vary from this maximum depending upon availability of data.
[b]Significance of beta weight associated with interaction term.
[c]Multiple correlation with all main effects and this interaction entered.
†$p < .10$; *$p < .05$; **$p < .01$; ***$p < .001$.

APPENDIX TABLE 6.7. Multiple Regressions: Significance of Interaction Terms in Analyses Involving Mothers' Work Status and Ways of Understanding and Peer Support Variables Predicting Adjustment for Boys

	Time 1 measures $(n = 62)^a$	Time 1 adjustment	Time 1 measures $(n = 62)^a$	Time 2 adjustment	Time 2 measures $(n = 43)^a$	Time 2 adjustment
	p^b	R^c	p^b	R^c	p^b	R^c
Psychological adjustment						
Perspective taking	**	.34†	***	.55**		
Person concepts						
Self-consciousness						
Internal locus of control					***	.53**
Friend activities					**	.44*
Sibling activities						
Illness						
Perspective taking	*	.32	**	.46**		
Person concepts			*	.34†		
Self-consciousness						
Internal locus of control					*	.32
Friend activities					*	.36†
Sibling activities						
Behavior problems (mother-rated)						
Perspective taking	**	.44*	***	.58***	†	.36†
Person concepts					*	.30
Self-consciousness			*	.39*		
Internal locus of control						
Friend activities	*	.40*				
Sibling activities						
Behavior problems (teacher-rated)						
Perspective taking			*	.45†		
Person concepts	†	.31	*	.44†		
Self-consciousness						
Internal locus of control						
Friend activities						
Sibling activities						

Note. Interpretations of interaction effects are provided in the text.
[a]n's vary from this maximum depending upon availability of data.
[b]Significance of beta weight associated with interaction term.
[c]Multiple correlation with all main effects and this interaction entered.
†$p < .10$; *$p < .05$; **$p < .01$; ***$p < .001$.

APPENDIX TABLE 6.8. Multiple Regressions: Significance of Interaction Terms in Analyses Involving Mothers' Work Status and Ways of Understanding and Peer Support Variables Predicting Adjustment for Girls

	Time 1 measures Time 1 adjustment $(n = 57)^a$		Time 1 measures Time 2 adjustment $(n = 57)^a$		Time 2 measures Time 2 adjustment $(n = 40)^a$	
	p^b	R^c	p^b	R^c	p^b	R^c
Psychological adjustment						
Perspective taking			*	.35		
Person concepts						
Self-consciousness					**	.42*
Internal locus of control					***	.49**
Friend activities			*	.55**	**	.47**
Sibling activities	*	.35†	**	.45*	*	.40*
Illness						
Perspective taking						
Person concepts						
Self-consciousness						
Internal locus of control					***	.80***
Friend activities			†	.36		
Sibling activities			*	.39†	**	.50**
Behavior problems (mother-rated)						
Perspective taking						
Person concepts						
Self-consciousness					***	.86***
Internal locus of control						
Friend activities	*	.42*				
Sibling activities						
Behavior problems (teacher-rated)						
Perspective taking						
Person concepts						
Self-consciousness			*	.61*		
Internal locus of control			*	.51*		
Friend activities						
Sibling activities					***	.74***

Note. Interpretations of interaction effects are provided in the text.
[a]n's vary from this maximum depending upon availability of data.
[b]Significance of beta weight associated with interaction term.
[c]Multiple correlation with all main effects and this interaction entered.
†$p < .10$; *$p < .05$; **$p < .01$; ***$p < .001$.

APPENDIX TABLE 6.9. Multiple Regressions: Significance of Interaction Terms in Analyses Involving Recent Changes and Ways of Understanding and Peer Support Variables Predicting Adjustment for Boys

	Time 1 measures Time 1 adjustment $(n = 62)^a$		Time 1 measures Time 2 adjustment $(n = 62)^a$		Time 2 measures Time 2 adjustment $(n = 46)^a$	
	p^b	R^c	p^b	R^c	p^b	R^c
Psychological adjustment						
Perspective taking	***	.95***	***	.77***		
Person concepts						
Self-consciousness						
Internal locus of control						
Friend activities						
Sibling activities	†	.23				
Illness						
Perspective taking	*	.36†				
Person concepts					*	.36†
Self-consciousness						
Internal locus of control						
Friend activities					*	.39*
Sibling activities						
Behavior problems (mother-rated)						
Perspective taking	***	.46**	**	.40*		
Person concepts						
Self-consciousness						
Internal locus of control						
Friend activities						
Sibling activities						
Behavior problems (teacher-rated)						
Perspective taking						
Person concepts	*	.43†				
Self-consciousness						
Internal locus of control						
Friend activities						
Sibling activities						

Note. Interpretations of interaction effects are provided in the text.
^{a}n's vary from this maximum depending upon availability of data.
^{b}Significance of beta weight associated with interaction term.
^{c}Multiple correlation with all main effects and this interaction entered.
$^†p < .10$; $^*p < .05$; $^{**}p < .01$; $^{***}p < .001$.

APPENDIX TABLE 6.10. Multiple Regressions: Significance of Interaction Terms in Analyses Involving Recent Changes and Ways of Understanding and Peer Support Variables Predicting Adjustment for Girls

	Time 1 measures / Time 1 adjustment $(n = 58)^a$		Time 1 measures / Time 2 adjustment $(n = 58)^a$		Time 2 measures / Time 2 adjustment $(n = 52)^a$	
	p^b	R^c	p^b	R^c	p^b	R^c
Psychological adjustment						
Perspective taking						
Person concepts						
Self-consciousness						
Internal locus of control						
Friend activities						
Sibling activities						
Illness						
Perspective taking						
Person concepts						
Self-consciousness	†	.28				
Internal locus of control						
Friend activities	*	.36†				
Sibling activities						
Behavior problems (mother-rated)						
Perspective taking					***	.66***
Person concepts					†	.43*
Self-consciousness	*	.32	*	.39†	**	.66***
Internal locus of control					***	.57**
Friend activities	†	.32				
Sibling activities						
Behavior problems (teacher-rated)						
Perspective taking						
Person concepts			*	.36		
Self-consciousness						
Internal locus of control						
Friend activities						
Sibling activities						

Note. Interpretations of interaction effects are provided in the text.
[a] n's vary from this maximum depending upon availability of data.
[b] Significance of beta weight associated with interaction term.
[c] Multiple correlation with all main effects and this interaction entered.
† $p < .10$; * $p < .05$; ** $p < .01$; *** $p < .001$.

APPENDIX TABLE 7.1. Pearson Correlations between Mothers' Adjustment and Children's Adjustment Measures

| | Mothers' adjustment | | | |
| | Relationships at Time 1 | | Relationships at Time 2 | |
	Psychological adjustment	Illness	Psychological adjustment	Illness
All children (*n* = 112)[a]				
Psychological adjustment	.10	−.21*	.16	−.17
Illness	−.04	.19	−.20	.25*
Behavior problems (mother-rated)	−.37***	.21*	−.30**	.22*
Behavior problems (teacher-rated)	.08	.19	−.27*	.14
Girls only (*n* = 54)[a]				
Psychological adjustment	.20	−.16	.20	−.35*
Illness	−.12	.26	−.28	.25
Behavior problems (mother-rated)	−.41***	.29	−.29	.22
Behavior problems (teacher-rated)	.09	.09	−.32	.09
Boys only (*n* = 58)[a]				
Psychological adjustment	.03	.07	.10	.05
Illness	.02	.25	−.04	.30*
Behavior problems (mother-rated)	−.34*	.27	−.37**	.21
Behavior problems (teacher-rated)	.10	.03	−.31	.30

Note. High scores on psychological adjustment signify better adjustment. Low score on illness and behavior problems (mother- and teacher-rated) signify better adjustment.

[a]*n*'s vary from this maximum depending upon availability of data.

*p < .05; **p < .01; ***p < .001.

APPENDIX TABLE 7.2. Pearson Correlations Between Relationship Quality and Children's and Mothers' Adjustment

	Relationship quality			
	Girls		Boys	
	Self-report $(n = 54)^a$	Observation $(n = 31)^a$	Self-report $(n = 59)^a$	Observation $(n = 31)^a$
Time 1 adjustment				
Children				
Psychological adjustment	.44*	.22	.25	.25
Illness	−.29	−.29	.04	.07
Behavior problems (mother-rated)	−.42**	−.11	−.53***	−.30
Behavior problems (teacher-rated)	−.32	−.08	−.16	.21
Mothers				
Psychological adjustment	.31*	.19	.27	.21
Illness	.01	−.24	−.21	−.07
Time 2 adjustment				
Children				
Psychological adjustment	−.05	.11	.20	.18
Illness	−.13	.09	.19	.15
Behavior problems (mother-rated)	−.39*	.05	−.54***	−.09
Behavior problems (teacher-rated)	.23	.28	−.32	.25
Mothers				
Psychological adjustment	.19	−.06	.19	.10
Illness	−.14	−.19	−.01	−.26

Note. High scores on psychological adjustment signify better adjustment. Low scores on illness and behavior problems (mother- and teacher-rated) signify better adjustment.

$^a n$'s vary from this maximum depending upon availability of data.

*$p < .05$; **$p < .01$; ***$p < .001$.

APPENDIX TABLE 7.3. Multiple Regressions for Relationship Quality and Adjustment, Time 1

Time 1 adjustment measure	R^2	Relationship quality Time 1 beta ($n = 59$)	
		Self-report	Observation
Children			
Psychological adjustment	.11***	.28**	.10
Illness	.02	−.08	−.07
Behavior problems (mother-rated)	.25***	−.54***	.13
Behavior problems (teacher-rated)	.14**.	−.38**	.34**
Mothers			
Psychological adjustment	.08**	.24*	.08
Illness	.03	−.07	−.13

Note. High scores on psychological adjustment signify better adjustment. Low scores on illness and behavior problems (mother- and teacher-rated) signify better adjustment.
*$p < .05$; **$p < .01$; ***$p < .001$.

APPENDIX TABLE 7.4. Multiple Regressions for Relationships Quality and Adjustment, Time 2

Time 2 adjustment measure	R^2	Relationship quality Time 2 beta ($n = 47$)	
		Self-report	Observation
Children			
Psychological adjustment	.02	.05	.11
Illness	.02	−.01	.14
Behavior problems (mother-rated)	.25***	−.52***	.16
Behavior problems (teacher-rated)	.11*	−.21	.31*
Mothers			
Psychological adjustment	.04	.20	−.08
Illness	.04	−.02	−.19

Note. High scores on psychological adjustment signify better adjustment. Low score on illness and behavior problems (mother- and teacher-rated) signify better adjustment.
*$p < .05$; ***$p < .001$.

APPENDIX TABLE 7.5. Multiple Regressions for Time 1 Relationship Quality and Time 2 Adjustment

		Relationship quality Time 1 beta ($n = 59$)	
Time 2 adjustment measure	R^2	Self-report	Observation
Children			
Psychological adjustment	.04	.08	.15
Illness	.02	−.14	.14
Behavior problems (mother-rated)	.37***	−.68***	.38**
Behavior problems (teacher-rated)	.09*	−.33*	.18
Mothers			
Psychological adjustment	.08*	.29*	−.06
Illness	.05	−.08	−.17

Note. High scores on psychological adjustment signify better adjustment. Low scores on illness and behavior problems (mother- and teacher-rated) signify better adjustment.
*$p < .05$; ***$p < .001$.

APPENDIX TABLE 7.6. Multiple Regressions for Dyad Links to Relationship Quality, Time 1

	Relationship quality ($n = 59$)	
	Self-report	Observation
r^2	.14†	−.24*
Mother–father conflict	−.03	.22
Mother–father closeness	−.05	−.04
Father–child conflict	.11	.28*
Father–child closeness	−.05	−.12
Loyalty strain	−.17	−.07
Mother extrafamilial involvement	.22*	.21
Child extrafamilial involvement	.11	.08

Note. Positive scores indicate good relationship quality.
†$p < .10$; *$p < .05$.

APPENDIX TABLE 7.7. Multiple Regressions for Family Links to Relationship Quality, Time 2

	Relationship quality ($n = 47$)	
	Self-report	Observation
r^2	.19***	−.07
SES	−.22*	.26†
Family stress	−.17†	−.02
Sibling adjustment	.40***	.02

Note. Positive scores indicate good relationship quality.
†$p < .10$; *$p < .05$; ***$p < .001$.

APPENDIX TABLE 8.1. Intercorrelations of Conflict Variables (Mothers)

	CTS reasoning	CTS violence	Husband violent	Legal conflict (Time 1)	Legal conflict (Time 2)	Interpersonal conflict (Time 1)	Interpersonal conflict (Time 2)
CTS violent	-.23*						
Husband violent	-.12	.55***					
Legal conflict (Time 1)	-.05	.15	.23*				
Legal conflict (Time 2)	-.09	.01	.12	.75***			
Interpersonal conflict (Time 1)	-.10	.17	.09	.27**	.23*		
Interpersonal conflict (Time 2)	-.09	.22*	.02	.16	.22*	.19	
Divorce settled (Time 2)	.25*	-.10	-.01	-.10	-.11	-.05	-.28**

Note. Overall $n = 120$ (Time 1), 97 (Time 2); n's for individual correlations vary due to incomplete data.
*$p < .05$; **$p < .01$; ***$p < .001$.

APPENDIX TABLE 8.2. Intercorrelations of Conflict Variables (Fathers)

	CTS reasoning	CTS violence	Legal conflict (Time 1)	Legal conflict (Time 2)	Interpersonal conflict (Time 1)	Interpersonal conflict (Time 2)
CTS violence	-.17					
Legal conflict (Time 1)	.30	.38				
Legal conflict (Time 2)	.05	.51*	.80***			
Interpersonal conflict (Time 1)	-.17	.27	.33	.39*		
Interpersonal conflict (Time 2)	.10	.03	-.03	-.12	.37	
Divorce settled (Time 2)	.15	-.08	-.29	-.10	-.38*	-.48**

Note. Overall $n = 57$ (Time 1), 46 (Time 2); n's for individual correlations vary due to incomplete data.
*$p < .05$; **$p < .01$; ***$p < .001$.

APPENDIX TABLE 8.3. Correlations between Conflict and Adjustment, All Children

	Self-report		Mother report				Teacher report	
	Psychological adjustment		Illness		Behavior problems		Behavior problems	
Conflict variable (source)	Time 1	Time 2	Time 1	Time 2	Time 1	Time 2	Time 1	Time 2
Time 1								
CTS (mother questionnaire)								
Reasoning							.25†	
Violence								.33*
Husband violent (mother report)					.20†		.25*	
Legal motions (court records)					.23*	.23*	.25*	
Vacating/restraining motions					.20*	.23*	.32**	
Custody motions								
Interpersonal conflict (family report)			.18†					
Time 2								
Legal motions (court records)								
Vacating/restraining motions								
Custody motions								
Interpersonal conflict (family report)		−.22*						.26*

Note. Overall $n = 120$ (Time 1), 97 (Time 2); n's for individual correlations vary due to incomplete data.
†$p < .10$; *$p < .05$; **$p < .01$.

APPENDIX TABLE 8.4. Correlations between Conflict and Children's Adjustment, Age and Sex Groups

Conflict variable (source)	Self-report		Mother report				Teacher report	
	Psychological adjustment		Illness		Behavior problems		Behavior problems	
	Time 1	Time 2	Time 1	Time 2	Time 1	Time 2	Time 1	Time 2
Time 1								
CTS (mother questionnaire)								
Reasoning		.49*	-.42*					-.48*
Violence								.60*
Husband violent (mother report)			.48*	.45*			-.48*	
Legal motions (court records)			.51*			.43**	.54*	
Vacating/restraining motions				.41*				
Custody motions	-.43*		-.40*			.41**	.49*, -.49*	
Interpersonal conflict (family report)			.49*	.54*				
Time 2								
Legal motions (court records)				.42*		.47**		
Vacating/restraining motions								
Custody motions						.43*		
Interpersonal conflict (family report)		-.39*, -.55**						

Note. Results appear in *italics* for boys 6–8 ($n = 29$ at Time 1), in **bold italics** for *boys 9–12* ($n = 33$), in regular type for girls 6–8 ($n = 30$), and in **bold type for girls 9–12** ($n = 28$).
*$p < .05$; **$p < .01$.

APPENDIX TABLE 8.5. Correlations between Conflict and Children's Time 2 Adjustment, by Status of Parents' Divorce (Settled vs. Not Settled by Time 2)

Conflict variable (source)	Self-report Psychological adjustment		Mother report Illness		Mother report Behavior problems		Teacher report Behavior problems	
	Settled	Not	Settled	Not	Settled	Not	Settled	Not
Time 1								
CTS (mother questionnaire)								
Reasoning	.37*							
Violence								.59**
Husband violent (mother report)								
Legal motions (court records)						.41**		
Vacating/restraining motions		−.36*				.41**		
Custody motions								
Interpersonal conflict (family report)								
Time 2								
Legal motions (court records)						.37*		
Vacating/restraining motions		−.40**				.42**		
Custody motions								
Interpersonal conflict (family report)	−.25†							.35†

Note. Overall $n = 51$ (settled), 46 (not settled); n's for individual correlations vary due to incomplete data.
†$p < .10$; *$p < .05$; **$p < .01$.

APPENDIX TABLE 8.6. Correlations between Conflict and Mothers' Adjustment

	Self-report			
	Psychological adjustment		Illness	
Conflict variable (source)				
Time 1	Time 1	Time 2	Time 1	Time 2
CTS (Mother questionnaire)				
Reasoning	.21*		−.24*	
Violence				
Husband violent (mother report)				
Legal motions (court records)				
Child-related motions^a	−.19*	*−.30**		
Interpersonal conflict (family report)				.23*
Time 2				
Legal motions (court records)				
Child-related motions^a		*−.31**		*.27*, .38**
Interpersonal conflict (family report)		−.30*		

Note. Results appear in regular type for all mothers ($n = 120$ at Time 1, 97 at Time 2), in **bold type** for mothers with **divorce settled by Time 2** ($n = 51$), and in *bold italics* for mothers with *divorce not settled by Time 2* ($n = 46$).

^aMotions regarding support, custody, and/or visitation.

*$p < .05$; **$p < .01$.

APPENDIX TABLE 8.7. Correlations between Predictor and Parental Conflict Variables

	CTS		Mother	Legal						Family	
				Total motions		Vacating/restraining		Child-related		Interpersonal conflict	
Predictor variable	Reasoning	Violence	Husband violent	Time 1	Time 2	Time 1	Time 2	Time 1	Time 2	Time 1	Time 2
Individual											
Spouse blame		.44***	.50***	.18*	.22*	.19*	.19*			.41*	
Self-blame						−.18*					
Trouble with necessities									.19*		
Family											
Parental substance abuse and/or violence		.40*** **.59****				.21*	.25**				
Couple											
Previous marriage			.26**								
Years married without children	.22*	−.23*									
Spouse job status higher	.21*			.46*			.46*			−.20*	
Wife changed status	.22*			.46*			.46*				
Coparenting Time 1			−.24**	−.54**	−.24**	−.43*	−.40*	−.59***		−.25**	
Coparenting Time 2					−.51**				−.51**	−.52**	
Mutual plans		−.31** **−.52***	−.24**		−.29**		−.24**	−.43*	−.40*	−.40*	−.46***

Notes. Results appear in regular type for mothers (*n* = 120 at Time 1, 97 at Time 2) and in **bold type for fathers** (*n* = 57 at Time 1, 46 at Time 2).
*p < .05; **p < .01; ***p < .001.

APPENDIX TABLE 10.1. Predicting Mothers' Adjustment from Custodial Household Variables

Family variables	Standardized regression coefficients predicting psychological adjustment	
	Within Time 1	Over time
Cohesion		−.27**
Companionship		
Openness to feedback	.21*	
Material resources	.22*	
Regular routines		
Safety concerns	−.22*	
Dyadic closeness		
Dyadic conflict		
Role flexibility		.32*
R	.39*	.41*
df	9,103	9,78

*p < .05; **p < .01.

APPENDIX TABLE 10.2. Predicting Mothers' Adjustment from Noncustodial Household Variables

Noncustodial household variables	Standardized regression coefficients predicting within Time 1	
	Psychological adjustment	Illness
Father–child closeness		
Father–child conflict		
Mother–father closeness	.21*	
Ease of arranging visits		
Frequency of visits		
Regularity of visits		
Loyalty strains		−.23†
R	.39*	.33
df	8,104	8,80

†p < .10; *p < .05.

APPENDIX TABLE 10.3a. Predicting Children's Adjustment from Custodial Household Variables within Time 1

Family variables	Standardized regression coefficients predicting adjustment within Time 1		
	Psychological adjustment	Illness	Behavior problems
Cohesion	−.21*		
Companionship			
Openness to feedback			
Material resources			−.30*
Regular routines			
Safety concerns			.20*
Dyadic closeness	.24		
Dyadic conflict		.19†	.26**
Role flexibility			
Age			
Sex		.21†	−.18†
R	.37	.31	.52**
df	11,108	11,93	11,92

†$p < .10$; * $p < .05$; **$p < .01$.

APPENDIX TABLE 10.3b. Predicting Children's Adjustment from Custodial Household Variables over Time

Family variables	Standardized regression coefficients predicting adjustment over time		
	Psychological adjustment	Illness	Behavior problems
Cohesion			
Companionship			
Openness to feedback			
Material resources			−.24*
Regular routines			
Safety concerns			.31*
Dyadic closeness	.21†		
Dyadic conflict			
Role flexibility			
Age	.20†	.20†	
Sex		.25*	−.20†
R	.36	.35	.49**
df	11,83	11,85	11,84

†$p < .10$; * $p < .05$; **$p < .01$.

APPENDIX TABLE 10.4a. Predicting Children's Adjustment from Noncustodial Household Variables within Time 1

Noncustodial household variables	Standardized regression coefficients predicting adjustment within Time 1		
	Psychological adjustment	Illness	Behavior problems
Father–child closeness		−.23*	
Father–child conflict			
Mother–father closeness			
Mother–father conflict		.33*	
Ease of arranging visits			
Frequency of visits			
Regularity of visits			
Loyalty strains	−.24*		.24*
Age			
Sex		.27**	−.20†
R	.26	.45**	.36
df	10,109	10,94	10,93

†$p < .10$; * $p < .05$; **$p < .01$.

APPENDIX TABLE 10.4b. Predicting Children's Adjustment from Noncustodial Household Variables over Time

Noncustodial household variables	Standardized regression coefficients predicting adjustment over time		
	Psychological adjustment	Illness	Behavior problems
Father–child closeness			
Father–child conflict		.20†	
Mother–father closeness			
Mother–father conflict			
Ease of arranging visits			
Frequency of visits			
Regularity of visits			
Loyalty strains			.29*
Age	.21†		
Sex		.21†	
R	.31	.34	.38
df	10,84	10,86	10,85

†$p < .10$; *$p < .05$.

APPENDIX TABLE 10.4c. Predicting Children's Adjustment from Noncustodial Household Variables within Time 2

Noncustodial household variables	Standardized regression coefficients predicting adjustment within Time 2		
	Psychological adjustment	Illness	Behavior problems
Father–child closeness		$-.25^\dagger$	
Father–child conflict			
Mother–father closeness			
Mother–father conflict			
Ease of arranging visits			
Frequency of visits			
Regularity of visits			
Loyalty strains	$-.31^*$		$.26^*$
Age			
Sex		$.26^*$	
R	$.43^\dagger$	$.35$	$.36$
df	10,84	10,86	10,85

$^\dagger p < .10; {}^* p < .05.$

APPENDIX TABLE 10.5. Predicting Family Social Integration from Custodial Household Variables

Family variables	Standardized regression coefficients		
	Within Time 1	Over time	Within Time 2
Cohesion	$-.16^\dagger$	$.18^\dagger$	
Companionship			$.27^{**}$
Openness to feedback	$-.18^\dagger$		$.40^{***}$
Material resources	$.16^\dagger$		
Regular routine			
Safety concerns			$-.30^*$
Dyadic closeness	$.18^\dagger$	$.22^*$	$.17^\dagger$
Dyadic conflict		$-.21^*$	
Role flexibility			
R	$.35^\dagger$	$.47^{**}$	$.53^{***}$
df	9,111	9,100	9,100

$^\dagger p < .10; {}^* p < .05; {}^{**} p < .01; {}^{***} p < .001.$

References

Abramson, J. H., Terepolsky, L., Brook, J. G., & Kark, S. L. (1965). Cornell Medical Index as a health measure in epidemiological studies: A test of the validity of a health questionnaire. *British Journal of Preventive Medicine, 19,* 102–110.

Achenbach, T. (1978). The Child Behavior Profile: I. Boys aged 6–11. *Journal of Consulting and Clinical Psychology, 46,* 478–483.

Achenbach, T., & Edelbrock, C. S. (1978). The Child Behavior Profile: II. Boys aged 12–16 and girls aged 6–11 and 12–16. *Journal of Consulting and Clinical Psychology, 47,* 223–233.

Achenbach, T., & Edelbrock, C. S. (1981). Behavioral problems and competencies reported by parents of normal and disturbed children aged four through sixteen. *Monographs of the Society for Research in Child Development, 46*(1, Serial No. 188).

Achenbach, T. M., Verhulst, F. C., Baron, G. D., & Althaus, M. (1987). A comparison of syndromes derived from the Child Behavior Checklist for American and Dutch boys aged 6–11. *Journal of Child Psychology and Psychiatry, 28,* 437–453.

Ahrons, C. R. (1979). The binuclear family: Two households, one family. *Alternative Lifestyles, 2,* 533–540.

Ahrons, C. R. (1980). Divorce: A crisis of family transition and change. *Family Relations, 29,* 533–540.

Ahrons, C. R. (1987). *Divorced families: A multidisciplinary developmental view.* New York: Norton.

Ahrons, C. R. (1995). *The good divorce.* New York: Harper.

Ahrons, C. R., & Wallisch, L. (1987). Parenting in the binuclear family: Relationships bewteen biological and stepparents. In K. Pasley & M. Ihinger-Tallman (Eds.), *Remarriage and stepparenting: Current research and theory* (pp. 225–256). New York: Guilford Press.

Allen, K. R. (1993). The dispassionate discourse of children's adjustment to divorce. *Journal of Marriage and the Family, 55,* 46–50.

Amato, P. R., & Keith, B. (1991). Parental divorce and the well-being of children: A meta-analysis. *Psychological Bulletin, 110,* 26–46.

Bateson, G. (1971). *Steps to an ecology of mind.* New York: Ballantine.

Bernard, J. (1972). *The future of marriage.* New York: World.

Block, J. H. (1965). *The Child-Rearing Practices Report.* Mimeograph, Institute of Human Development, University of California, Berkeley.

Block, J. H. (1984). *Sex role identity and ego development.* San Francisco: Jossey-Bass.

Block, J. H., Block, J., & Gjerde, P. F. (1986). The personality of children prior to divorce: A prospective study. *Child Development, 57,* 827–840.

Block, J. H., Block, J., & Morrison, A. (1981). Parental agreement–disagreement on child-rearing orientations and gender-related personality correlates in children. *Child Development, 52,* 965–974.

Bohannon, P. (1970). The six stations of divorce. In P. Bohannon (Ed.), *Divorce and after* (pp. 29–55). New York: Doubleday.

Bowen, M. (1978). *Family therapy in clinical practice.* New York: Jason Aronson.

Bray, J. H., Berger, S. H., Silverblatt, A. H., & Hollier, A. (1987). Family process and organization during early remarriage: A preliminary analysis. In J. P. Vincent (Ed.), *Advances in family intervention, assessment and theory* (Vol. 4, pp. 253–280). Greenwich, CT: JAI Press.

Brown, R., & Kulik, J. (1977). Flashbulb memories. *Cognition, 5,* 73–99.

Bursik, K. (1986). *Adaptation to marital separation and divorce: A context for ego development in adult women.* Unpublished doctoral dissertation, Boston University.

Bursik, K. (1991). Adaptation to divorce and ego development in adult women. *Journal of Personality and Social Psychology, 60,* 300–306.

Camara, K. A., & Resnick, G. (1987). The interaction between marital and parental subsystems in mother-custody, father-custody and two-parent households: Effects on children's social development. In J. P. Vincent (Ed.), *Advances in family intervention, assessment and theory* (Vol. 4, pp. 165–196) Greenwich, CT: JAI Press.

Camara, K. A., & Resnick, G. (1989). Styles of conflict resolution and cooperation between divorced parents: Effects on child behavior and adjustment. *American Journal of Orthopsychiatry, 59,* 560–575.

Chodorow, N. (1978). *The reproduction of mothering.* Berkeley: University of California Press.

Copeland, A. P. (1984). An early look at divorce: Mother–child interactions in the first post-separation year. *Journal of Divorce, 8,* 17–30.

Copeland, A. P. (1985a). Individual differences in children's reactions to divorce. *Journal of Clinical Child Psychology, 14,* 11–19.

Copeland, A. P. (1985b). Self-control ratings and mother–child interaction. *Journal of Clinical Child Psychology, 14,* 124–131.

Copeland, A. P. (1990). Behavioral differences in the interactions between Type A and B mothers and their children. *Behavioral Medicine, 16,* 111–117.

Cowan, P. A., & Cowan, C. P. (1992). *When partners become parents: The big life change for couples.* New York: Basic Books.

Crandall, V. C., Katkovsky, J., & Crandall, V. J. (1965). Children's beliefs in their own control of reinforcements in intellectual–academic achievement situations. *Child Development, 36,* 91–109.

Crosby, F. (1990). Divorce and work life among women managers. In H. Y. Grossman

& N. L. Chester (Eds.), *The meaning and experience of work in women's lives* (pp. 121–142). Hillsdale, NJ: Erlbaum.

Dornbusch, S. M., Carlsmith, J. M., Bushwall, S. J., Ritter, P. L., Leiderman, H., Hastorf, A. H., & Gross, Ruth T. (1985). Single parents, extended households, and the control of adolescents. *Child Development, 56,* 326–341.

Dornbusch, S. M., & Gray, K. D. (1988). Single-parent families. In S. M. Dornbusch & M. H. Strober (Eds.), *Feminism, children, and the new families* (pp. 274–296). New York: Guilford Press.

Edelbrock, C. S., & Achenbach, T. M. (1984). The Teacher Version of the Child Behavior Profile: I. Boys aged 6–11. *Journal of Consulting and Clinical Psychology, 52*(2), 207–217.

Emery, R. E. (1982). Interparental conflict and the children of discord and divorce. *Psychological Bulletin, 92,* 310–330.

Emery, R. E. (1988). *Marriage, divorce, and children's adjustment.* Newbury Park, CA: Sage.

Fincham, F. D., Grych, J. H., & Osborne, L. N. (1994). Does marital conflict cause child maladjustment? Directions and challenges for longitudinal research. *Journal of Family Psychology, 8,*(2), 128–140.

Furstenberg, F. F., & Cherlin, A. J. (1991). *Divided families.* Cambridge, MA: Harvard University Press.

Gilligan, C. (1982). *In a different voice.* Cambridge, MA: Harvard University Press.

Glick, P.C. (1979). *The future of the American family.* Washington, DC: Bureau of the Census, Current Population Reports Special Studies.

Golan, N. (1983). *Passing through transitions: A guide for practitioners.* New York: Free Press.

Gove, W. (1978). Sex differences in mental illness among adult men and women: An examination of four questions raised regarding whether or not women actually have higher rates. *Social Science and Medicine, 12,* 187–198.

Gurin, G., Veroff, J., & Feld, S. (1960). *Americans view their mental health.* New York: Basic Books.

Guttmann, J., Geva, N., & Gefen, S. (1988). Teachers' and school children's stereotypic perception of the 'child of divorce.' *American Educational Research Journal, 25,* 555–571.

Harter, S. (1982). The Perceived Competence Scale for Children. *Child Development, 53,* 87–97.

Healy, J. M., Jr., Malley, J. M., & Stewart, A. J. (1990). Children and their fathers after parental separation. *American Journal of Orthopsychiatry, 60*(4), 531–543.

Healy, J. M., Jr., Stewart, A. J., & Copeland, A. P. (1993). The role of self-blame in children's adjustment to parental separation. *Personality and Social Psychology Bulletin, 19,* 279–289.

Hetherington, E. M. (1979). Divorce: A child's perspective. *American Psychologist, 34,* 851–858.

Hetherington, E. M. (1987). Family relations six years after divorce. In K. Pasley & M. Ihinger-Tallman (Eds.), *Remarriage and stepparenting: Current research and theory* (pp. 185–205). New York: Guilford Press.

Hetherington, E. (1989). Coping with family transitions: Winners, losers, and survivors. *Child Develoment, 60*(1), 1–14.

Hetherington, E. M., & Arasteh, J.D. (1988). *Impact of divorce, single parenting, and stepparenting on children.* Hillsdale, NJ: Erlbaum.

Hetherington, E. M., Cox, M., & Cox, R. (1977). Beyond father absence: Conceptualizations of the effects of divorce. In E. M. Hetherington & R. D. Parke (Eds.), *Contemporary readings in child psychology* (pp. 308–315). New York: McGraw-Hill.

Hetherington, E. M., Cox, M., & Cox, R. (1982). Effects of divorce on parents and children. In M.E. Lamb (Ed.), *Nontraditional families: Parenting and child development* (pp. 233–288). Hillsdale, NJ: Erlbaum.

Hochschild, A. (1989). *The second shift.* New York: Viking.

Hollingshead, A. B., & Redlich, F. C. (1958). *Social class and mental illness.* New York: Wiley.

Johnston, J. R. (1993). Family transitions and children's functioning: The case of parental conflict and divorce. In P. A. Cowan, D. Field, D. A. Hansen, A. Skolnick, & G. E. Swanson (Eds.), *Family, self, and society: Toward a new agenda for family research* (pp. 197–234). Hillsdale, NJ: Erlbaum.

Johnston, J. R., Kline, M., & Tachann, J. M. (1989). Ongoing postdivorce conflict: Effects on children of joint custody and frequent access. *American Journal of Orthopsychiatry, 59,* 577–592.

Kalter, N. (1990). *Growing up with divorce: Helping your child avoid immediate and later emotional problems.* New York: Free Press.

Kitson, G. C. (1992). *Portrait of divorce: Adjustment to marital breakdown.* New York: Guilford Press.

Koestner, R., & McClelland, D.C. (1992). The affiliation motive. In C.P. Smith (Ed.), *Motivation and personality: Handbook of thematic content analysis* (pp. 205–210). New York: Cambridge University Press

Krantz, S. E. (1988). Divorce and children. In S. M. Dornbusch & M. H. Strober (Eds.), *Feminism, children, and the new families* (pp. 249–273). New York: Guilford Press.

Kulka, R. A., & Weingarten, H. (1979). The long-term effects of parental divorce in childhood on adult adjustment. *Journal of Social Issues, 35,* 50–78.

Kurdek, L. (1987). Children's adjustment to divorce: An ecological perspective. In J. P. Vincent (Ed.), *Advances in family intervention, assessment and theory* (Vol. 4, pp. 1–31). Greenwich, CT: JAI Press.

Kurz, D. (1995). *For richer, for poorer: Mothers confront divorce.* New York: Routledge.

Lidz, T. (1968). *The person: His development throughout the life cycle.* New York: Basic Books.

Lykes, M. B. (1985). Gender and individualistic vs. collectivist bases for notions about the self. In A. J. Stewart & M. B. Lykes (Eds.), *Gender and personality: Current perspectives on theory and research* (pp. 268–295). Durham, NC: Duke University Press.

Markus, H., & Oyserman, D. (1989). Gender and thought: The role of the self-concept. In M. Crawford & M. Gentry (Eds.), *Gender and thought: Psychological perspectives* (pp. 100–127). New York: Springer-Verlag.

Mash, E. J., Terdal, L., & Anderson, K. (1973). The response–class matrix: A procedure for recording parent–child interactions. *Journal of Consulting and Clinical Psychology, 40,* 163–164.

McNair, D., Lorr, M., & Droppleman, L. (1971). *Profile of Mood States.* San Diego: Educational and Industrial Testing Service.

Miller, J. B. (1986). *Toward a new psychology of women.* Boston: Beacon.

Minuchin, S. (1974). *Families and family therapy.* Cambridge, MA: Harvard University Press.

Minuchin, S. (1984). *Family kaleidoscope.* Cambridge, MA: Harvard University Press.

Minuchin, S., Baker, L., Rosman, B. L., Liebman, R., Milman, L., & Todd, T. G. (1975). A conceptual model of psychosomatic illness in children: Family organization and family therapy. *Archives of General Psychiatry, 32,* 1031–1038.

Minuchin, S., Montalvo, B., Guerney, B. G., Rosman, B. L., & Schumer, F. (1967). *Families of the slums.* New York: Basic Books.

Minuchin, S., Rosman, B. L., & Baker, L. (1978) *Psychosomatic families: Anorexia nervosa in context.* Cambridge, MA: Harvard University Press.

National Center for Health Statistics. (1989). *Advance report of final divorce statistics, 1986* (Monthly Vital Statistics Report, Vol. 38, No. 2 [Suppl.], DHHS Publication No. PHS 90–1120). Hyattsville, MD: U.S. Public Health Service.

Norton, A. J., & Glick, P. C. (1979). Marital instability in America: Past, present and future. In G. Levinger & O. C. Moles (Eds.), *Divorce and separation* (pp. 6–19). New York: Basic Books.

Norton, A. J., & Glick, P. C. (1986). One-parent families: A social and economic profile. *Journal of Family Relations, 35,* 9–17.

Olson, D. H. (1977). Insiders' and outsiders' views of relationships: Research and strategies. In G. Levinger & H. Raush (Eds.), *Close relationships* (pp. 115–136). Amherst: University of Massachusetts Press.

Olson, D. H., Sprenkle, D. H., & Russell, C. S. (1979). Circumplex model of marital and family systems: I. Cohesion and adaptability dimensions, family types, and clinical applications. *Family Process, 18,* 3–27.

Parsons, T., & Bales, R. F. (1955). *Family, socialization and interaction process.* Glencoe, IL: Free Press.

Peevers, B. H., & Secord, P. F. (1973). Developmental changes in attribution of descriptive concepts to persons. *Journal of Personality and Social Psychology, 27,* 120–128.

Peterson, R. R. (1989). *Women, work, and divorce.* Albany: State University of New York Press.

Pillemer, D., Rhinehart, E. D., & White, S. H. (1986). Memories of life transitions: The first year in college. *Human Learning, 5,* 109–123.

Popenoe, D. (1993). American family decline: 1960–1990. *Journal of Marriage and the Family, 55,* 527–555.

Price, S. J., & McKenry, P. C. (1988). *Divorce.* Newbury Park, CA: Sage.

Pringle, M. K. (1974). *The needs of children.* New York: Schocken.

Raschke, H. J. (1987). Divorce. In M. B. Sussman & S. K. Steinmetz (Eds.), *Handbook of marriage and the family* (pp. 597–624). New York: Plenum Press.

Reiss, D. (1981). *The family's construction of reality.* Cambridge, MA: Harvard University Press.

Rice, J. K. (1994). Reconsidering research on divorce, family life cycle, and the meaning of family. *Psychology of Women Quarterly, 18,* 559–584.

Riessman, C. K. (1990). *Divorce talk: Women and men make sense of personal relationships.* New Brunswick, NJ: Rutgers University Press.

Robinson, J. P., Shaver, P., & Wrightsman, L.S. (1991). *Measures of personality and social psychological attitudes.* San Diego, CA: Academic Press.

Rosen, B. C., & D'Andrade, R. (1959). The psychosocial origins of achievement motivation. *Sociometry, 22,* 185–218.

Rosenberg, M. (1965). *Society and the adolescent self-image.* Princeton, NJ: Princeton University Press.

Rubin, D. (1986). Autobiographical memory. New York: Cambridge University Press.

Seligman, M., & Darling, R. B. (1997). *Ordinary families, special children: A systems approach to childhood disability* (2nd ed.). New York: Guilford Press.

Smith, C.P. (Ed.). (1992). *Motivation and personality: Handbook of thematic content analysis.* New York: Cambridge University Press.

Stacey, J. (1990). *Brave new families.* New York: Basic Books.

Stacey, J. (1991). Backward toward the postmodern family: Reflections on gender, kinship, and class in the Silicon Valley. In A. Wolfe (Ed.), *America at century's end* (pp. 17–34). Berkeley and Los Angeles: University of California Press.

Stannard, D. (1979). *Changes in the American family: Fiction and reality.* New Haven: Yale University Press.

Stewart, A. J. (1982). The course of individual adaptation to life changes. *Journal of Personality and Social Psychology, 42,* 1100–1113.

Stewart, A. J., & Chester, N. L. (1982). Sex differences in human motives: Achievement, affiliation and power. In A. J. Stewart (Ed.), *Motivation and society* (pp. 172–218). San Francisco: Jossey-Bass.

Stewart, A. J., & Healy, J. M., Jr. (1985). Personality and adaptation to life change. In R. Hogan & W. Jones (Ed.), *Perspectives on personality: Theory, measurement, and interpersonal dynamics* (pp. 117–144). Greenwich, CT: JAI Press.

Stewart, A. J., & Healy, J. M., Jr. (1992). Assessing adaptation to life changes in terms of psychological stances toward the environment. In C. P. Smith (Ed.), *Motivation and personality: Handbook of thematic content analysis* (pp. 440–450). New York: Cambridge University Press.

Stewart, A. J., & Rubin, Z. (1974). The power motive in the dating couple. *Journal of Personality and Social Psychology, 34,* 305–309.

Stewart, A. J., Sokol, M., Healy, J. M., Jr., & Chester, N. L. (1986). Longitudinal studies of psychological consequences of life changes in children and adults. *Journal of Personality and Social Psychology, 50,* 143–151.

Stewart, A. J., Sokol, M., Healy, J. M., Jr., Chester, N. L., & Weinstock-Savoy, D. (1982). Adaptation to life changes in children and adults: Cross-sectional studies. *Journal of Personality and Social Psychology, 43,* 1270–1281.

Straus, M. A. (1974). Leveling, civility, and violence in the family. *Journal of Marriage and the Family, 36,* 13–29 [also addendum, 36, 442–445].

Straus, M. A. (1979). Measuring intrafamily conflict and violence: The Conflict Tactics (CT) Scales. *Journal of Marriage and the Family, 41,* 75–88.

Talbot, N. B. (1976). *Raising children in modern America.* Boston: Little, Brown.

Thompson, L., & Walker, A. J. (1989). Gender in families: Women and men in marriage, work and parenthood. *Journal of Marriage and the Family, 51,* 845–871.

Thornton, A. (1989). Changing attitudes toward family issues in the U.S. *Journal of Marriage and the Family, 51,* 873–893.

Turk, D. C., & Kerns, R. D. (Eds.). (1985). *Health, illness and families: A life-span perspective.* New York: Wiley.

Veroff, J., Kulka, R. A., & Douvan, E. (1981). *Mental health in America.* New York: Basic Books.

Vincent, J. P. (Ed.). (1987). *Advances in family intervention, assessment and theory* (Vol. 4). Greenwich, CT: JAI Press.

Wahler, H. J. (1973). *Wahler Physical Symptoms Inventory.* Los Angeles: Western Psychological Services.

Walker, H. A. (1988). Black–white differences in marriage and family patterns. In S. M. Dornbusch, & M. H. Strober (Eds.), *Feminism, children, and the new families* (pp. 87–112). New York: Guilford Press.

Wallerstein, J. S., & Blakeslee, S. (1989). *Second chances.* New York: Ticknor & Fields.

Wallerstein, J. S., & Kelly, J. B. (1980). *Surviving the breakup.* New York: Basic.

Wechsler, D. (1974). *Manual for the Wechsler Intelligence Scale for Children, Revised.* New York: Psychological Corporation.

Weiss, R. (1975). *Marital separation.* New York: Basic Books.

Weitzman, L. J. (1985). *The divorce revolution.* New York: Free Press.

Weitzman, L. J. (1988). Women and children last: The social and economic consequences of divorce law reform. In S. M. Dornbusch, & M. H. Strober (Eds.), *Feminism, children, and the new families* (pp. 212–248). New York: Guilford Press.

White, K. M., Speisman, J. C., & Costos, D. (1983). Young adults and their parents: From individuation to maturity. *New Directions in Child Development, 22,* 61–76.

White, K. M., Speisman, J. C., Jackson, D., Bartis, S., & Costos, D. (1986). Intimacy maturity and its correlates in young married couples. *Journal of Personality and Social Psychology, 50,* 152–162.

Whitehead, B. D. (1993, April). Dan Quayle was right. *Atlantic Monthly,* pp. 47–84.

Winter, D. G. (1973). *The power motive.* New York: Free Press.

Winter, D .G. (1988). The power motive in women—and men. *Journal of Personality and Social Psychology, 54,* 510–519.

Winter, D. G. (1991). Measuring personality at a distance: Development of an integrated system for scoring motives in running text. In A. J. Stewart, J. M. Healy, Jr., & D. Ozer (Eds.), *Perspectives in personality: Approaches to understanding lives* (pp. 59–89). London: Jessica Kingsley.

Winter, D. G. (1992). Power motivation revisited. In C. P. Smith (Ed.), *Motivation and personality: Handbook of thematic content analysis* (pp. 301–310). New York: Cambridge University Press.

Winter, D. G., & Barenbaum, N. B. (1985). Responsibility and the power motive in women and men. *Journal of Personality, 53,* 335–355.

Zaslow, M. J. (1988). Sex differences in children's response to parental divorce: I. Research methodology and postdivorce family forms. *American Journal of Orthopsychiatry, 58,* 355–378.

Zaslow, M. (1989). Sex differences in children's response to parental divorce: II. Samples, variables, ages, and sources. *American Journal of Orthopsychiatry, 59,* 118–141.

Index

Page numbers in italics indicate reference entries.